Lipid Nutrition Guidelines

Harumi Okuyama, Sheriff Sultan, Naoki Ohara, Tomohito Hamazaki, Peter H Langsjoen, Rokuro Hama, Yoichi Ogushi, Tetsuyuki Kobayashi, Shunji Natori, Hajime Uchino, Yoko Hashimoto, Shiro Watanabe, Kenjiro Tatematsu, Daisuke Miyazawa, Mikio Nakamura and Kentaro Oh-hashi

Lipid Nutrition Guidelines: A Comprehensive Analysis

MDPI • Basel • Beijing • Wuhan • Barcelona • Belgrade • Manchester • Tianjin • Tokyo • Cluj

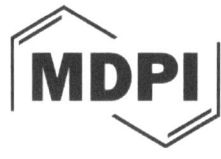

AUTHORS

PROF. EMERITUS HARUMI OKUYAMA
Nagoya City University, Nagoya; Visiting Scientist, Institute for Consumer Science and Human Life, Kinjo Gakuin University, Nagoya, Japan

PROF. SHERIF SULTAN
Vascular and Endovascular Surgery, National University of Ireland Galway; Chief, Vascular and Endovascular Surgery, University Hospital Galway & Galway Clinic; Chairman of Western Vascular Institute, Galway, Ireland; President, International Society for Vascular Surgery

PROF. NAOKI OHARA
College of Pharmacy, Kinjo Gakuin University, Nagoya, Japan

LATE PROF. EMERITUS TOMOHITO HAMAZAKI
University of Toyama, Toyama, Japan; Toyama Onsen Daini Hospital, Toyama, Japan

DR. PETER H LANGSJOEN
Clinical Cardiology Practice, Tyler, TX, USA

DR. ROKURO HAMA
NPO Japan Institute of Pharmacovigilance, Osaka, Japan; Osaka University School of Medicine, Osaka, Japan

PROF. EMERITUS YOICHI OGUSHI
Tokai University School of Medicine, Ogushi Institute of Medical Informatics, Hiratsuka, Japan

PROF. TETSUYUKI KOBAYASHI
Graduate School of Humanities and Sciences, Institute for Human Life Innovation, Ochanomizu University, Tokyo, Japan

PROF. EMERITUS SHUNJI NATORI
Faculty of Pharmaceutical Sciences, University of Tokyo, Tokyo, Japan

DR. HAJIME UCHINO
Medical Corporation Uchinokai, Kumamoto, Japan

DR. YOKO HASHIMOTO
Lecturer, Department of Biochemistry, School of Dentistry, Aichi-Gakuin University, Nagoya, Japan

ASSOC. PROF. SHIRO WATANABE
Institute of Natural Medicine, University of Toyama, Toyama, Japan

DR. KENJIRO TATEMATSU
Lecturer, Department of Radiochemistry, Gifu Pharmaceutical University, Gifu, Japan

ASSOC. PROF. DAISUKE MIYAZAWA
College of Pharmacy, Kinjo Gakuin University, Nagoya, Japan

DR. MIKIO NAKAMURA
NPO Global Network of Food Safety, Osaka, Japan

ASSOC. PROF. KENTARO OH-HASHI
Department of Chemistry and Biomolecular Science, Faculty of Engineering, Gifu University, Gifu, Japan

EDITORIAL OFFICE
MDPI
St. Alban-Anlage 66
Basel, Switzerland

For citation purposes, cite as indicated below:

Okuyama, H.; Sultan, S.; Ohara, N.; Hamazaki, T.; Langsjoen, P.H.; Hama, R.; Ogushi, T.; Kobayashi, T.; Natori, S.; Uchino, H.; Hashimoto, Y.; Watanabe, S.; Tatematsu, K.; Miyazawa, D.; Nakamura, M.; Oh-hashi, K. *Lipid Nutrition Guidelines: A Comprehensive Analysis*; MDPI: Basel, Switzerland, 2021.

ISBN 978-3-03943-945-4 (Hbk)
ISBN 978-3-03943-946-1 (PDF)

doi:10.3390/books978-3-03943-946-1

© 2021 by the author. The book is Open Access and distributed under the Creative Commons Attribution license (CC BY-NC-ND), which allows users to download, copy and build upon published work non-commercially, as long as the author and publisher are properly credited. If the material is transformed or built upon, the resulting work may not be distributed without permission from the authors.

Contents

About the First Author	ix
In Memory of Tomohito Hamazaki, Professor Emeritus, University of Toyama	xi
Preface	xiii
Acknowledgment	xv

CHAPTER 1
How the Cholesterol Hypothesis Lost Credibility: A Brief Summary — 1

1.1. Lipid Nutrition Based on the Cholesterol Hypothesis Is Risky	1
1.2. Pharmacological Mechanisms of Excess Linoleic Acid and Relative n-3 Deficiency Syndrome	4
1.3. Pharmacological Implications of the n-6/n-3 Balance of Dietary and Tissue Lipids	6
1.4. Essential Roles of the Arachidonic Acid Cascade	9
1.5. Anti-Inflammatory Hydroxylated Mediators Produced from EPA and DHA	9
1.6. Platelet-Activating Factor and Ethanol Amide of Fatty Acids (Anandamide)	11
1.7. Gene Technology Applied to Lipid Nutrition	13
1.8. Why Some Clinical Studies Have Failed to Show the Effectiveness of n-3 Lipids in Suppressing Allergic and Inflammatory Diseases	13
1.9. Critical Evaluation of the American Heart Association's Basis for Recommending Increased Intake of Vegetable Oils Instead of Animal Fats	15
Chapter 1 Summary	17

CHAPTER 2
All Mainstream Lipid Nutrition Guidelines Disregard Evidence That Some Types of Vegetable Fats and Oils Induce Stroke and Disrupt Endocrines — 19

2.1. Toxicity of Some Types of Vegetable Fats and Oils Observed in Stroke-Prone Spontaneously Hypertensive Rats	19
2.2. Mechanisms of Canola Oil and Hydrogenated Oil Causing Toxicity	22
2.3. Hydrogenation of Vegetable Oils Produces Hydrogenated Vitamin K1 (Dihydro-VKI) in Addition to Trans-fatty Acids, and Clinical Reports Correlate This Hydrogenation with the VK2–Osteocalcin Link	23
2.4. What Differences Could We Expect by Viewing Trans-Fat or Dihydro-ViK1 as a Health Risk?	26
Chapter 2 Summary	29

CHAPTER 3

Industry-Oriented Lipid Nutritional Guidelines Have Likely Endangered Some Populations — 31

3.1. Changes in Lipid Nutrition Are Consistent with Changes in Disease Patterns in Japan — 31
3.2. The People of Hisayama Town Were Misled by Nutritionists Unquestioningly Following the Mainstream Recommendations — 32
3.3. International Differences in Population and Health Status Are Potentially Associated with Lipid Nutrition — 34
3.4. Some Types of Vegetable Oils with Endocrine-Disrupting Activity Affect Sexual Development and Mental Disorders — 40
3.5 The Wrong Lipid Nutrition Is Potentially Endangering the Japanese People — 46
3.6 Additional Data Must Be Collected on the Intake of Different Types of Fats and Oils in Different Countries and Ethnic Groups — 48
Chapter 3 Summary — 49

CHAPTER 4

Comprehensive Risk Management in Light of Japan's Medical Care Act — 51

4.1. Cholesterol-Lowering Medications and the Medical Care Act — 52
4.2. Two Different Types of Guidelines for Hypertension, from Different Standpoints of the Medical Care Act — 56
4.3. Failure of Hypoglycemic Medicines to Demonstrate Reductions in All-Cause Mortality in Japan — 58
4.4. Comprehensive Risk Management: The Approach of the Japanese Society of Internal Medicine — 59

Epilogue — 65
Key Issues — 57
Notes Added in Proof — 69
References — 71

About the First Author

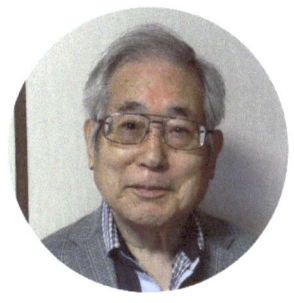

Harumi Okuyama received his Ph.D. from the University of Tokyo. He held the positions of Research Assistant at the University of Tokyo, Associated Professor and Professor at Nagoya City University (1972–2005), and Professor at the School of Pharmacy, Kinjo Gakuin University (–2012). He later returned to research as a visiting researcher at the Institute of Consumer Sciences and Human Life (2012–). During that time, he also served as a visiting professor at Baylor College of Medicine (Houston, TX), University of Illinois at Chicago (Chicago, IL), Dalian College of Medicine, Dalian University (Dalian, China), and The University of Toyama (Toyama, Japan).

Following his participation in the founding of the Japan Society for Lipid Nutrition, he served as the Society's first President. In this role and while continuing basic and clinical research into fats and oils, he strove to convey to the next generation the true information known about lipids and which oils were safe for consumption based on the latest evidence available. He also served as Chairman of the NGO Japan Council for the Safety Evaluation of Fats and Oils in Foods.

He started his research career as a graduate student of the University of Tokyo, focusing on identifying fatty acid synthetases as thermo-receptors to alter the chain length and/or the degree of unsaturation of fatty acids produced *in vitro* depending on the temperature in some microorganisms. Using animal models, he contributed to revealing the mechanisms of biosynthesis of membrane phospholipids with different fatty acids at the 1- and -2 positions. He then extended his research interests to estimating the nutritional values of various fatty acids. His group reached the following conclusions. (1) Plasma high cholesterol is a predictor of longevity. (2) Medicines to lower the LDL-C/HDL-C ratio do not bring about beneficial effects on atherosclerotic diseases when the objective endpoint of mortality is used. (3) The action mechanisms of statins involve the inhibition of isoprenyl intermediate formation and the inhibition of mitochondrial ATP generation. (4) In a stroke-prone rat model, certain types of common vegetable oils (e.g., canola, olive, and hydrogenated soybean oils) were found to accelerate cerebral bleeding, kidney inflammation, decreasing platelet counts, and decreasing tissue levels of testosterone. (5) These toxic oils share the same mechanism of action as statins and warfarin. (6) While some European countries have steadily increasing populations, many Mediterranean and East Asian countries, particularly Japan, are experiencing serious problems with decreasing birth rates and declining populations. Prof. Okuyama and his group have presented scientific evidence that the decreasing birth rate in Japan is correlated with increased intake of some types of vegetable oils, and thus the current, authoritative, mainstream lipid guidelines from the World Health Organization, backed by academics and industry-oriented people, are the major cause of the rapid decline in the Japanese population.

Alongside the coauthors of this work and other scientists and clinicians who acknowledge the scientific evidence available, Prof. Okuyama recommends restricting the intake of vegetable fats and oils demonstrated to have toxic effects in animal models and increasing the intake of cholesterol and animal fats to an extent that does not lead to obesity.

In Memory of Tomohito Hamazaki, Professor Emeritus, University of Toyama

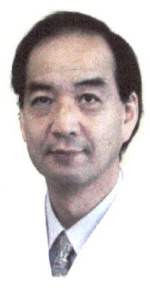

I lost my most reliable, irreplaceable comrade while we were finishing proofreading this book. Tomohito Hamazaki suffered an ischemic stroke in early September 2020 and did not come back to us. When young, we competed in lowering the plasma ARA/EPA balance, achieving similarly low ratios. As a clinician, he was totally committed to his patients, to the extent that he often took the medicines he prescribed just to confirm for himself their safety and effectiveness. I used to worry about the possible side effects of these drugs on him, but that's the kind of man he was.

In around 1992, we founded the Japan Society of Lipid Nutrition, and we fought together for over a quarter of century to revise the mainstream guidelines of lipid nutrition. Our first collaborative work was to send critical comments to the Japan Atherosclerosis Society arguing that, in order to help reveal the causal relationship between cholesterol and atherosclerosis, data for patients with familial hypercholesterolemia (FH) should be analyzed separately from those of general populations without FH. We sent similar comments to other medical societies, often without response. Inevitably, it fell to Professor Hamazaki to send these comments as lead author because I am a co-medical. Recently, we came to realize that the targets of our collaborative work are not the World Health Organization, medical societies, or the administrative authorities but rather hidden actors in the global pharma–food industry sectors that influence the direction that the WHO, medical societies, and the administrative authorities take.

In fact, these actors influence many aspects of medical care. Their involvement is often discussed in terms of a "necessary evil" that helps to provide the vast sums of money that medical care requires, although they even provide funds to some individual prescribers of medicines. As we discuss in this book, the relationships that now exist between these actors, clinicians, and the administrative authorities have gone beyond the permissible range, and the nation and individual patients are being hugely disadvantaged by this. Reflecting on our many discussions of this situation, I made up my mind to continue walking the difficult road that Professor Hamazaki and I started on together, fighting to secure patients' rights in view of Japan's Medical Care Act, rights that these complex relationships seem to threaten.

Professor Hamazaki had an extraordinary talent for foreign languages and a keen interest in the peoples that spoke them. As a clinician and former president of the Japan Society for Lipid Nutrition, he did much to advance our knowledge of nutrition to benefit the people of the world. He will be greatly missed.

Harumi Okuyama

Preface

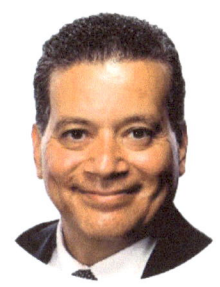

Professor Okuyama's books stand tall in a dark field muddied by greed and medical misadventures. His honesty and professionalism excel in painting the truth about atherosclerosis and its relation to high LDL-cholesterol.

Raising the proportion of polyunsaturated vegetable oils in place of saturated animal fats is recommended by the World Health Organization (WHO) and many authoritative societies which are supported by industry. I know that there are many observations against the polyunsaturated vegetable fats/animal fats balance theory, as I am an author of the book *Fats and Cholesterol Don't Cause Heart Attacks and Statins Are not The Solution* (Columbus Publishing, U.K., 2016), in which I re-evaluated the side effects of statin therapy.

Harumi Okuyama, Ph.D. and Professor Emeritus at Nagoya City University is unique in that he does not disregard data from animal experiments revealing the pharmacological mechanisms of statin actions and the effects of dietary fats and oils. He also brings together all lines of evidence from clinical observational studies that are consistent with these mechanisms. His group found toxic effects of common vegetable oils such as canola and hydrogenated vegetable fats. The animal experiments his group conducted are straightforward and reproducible. In fact, several laboratories from other countries, including Health Canada, confirm his group's findings.

The conclusions the authors discuss in detail here are sound: that accelerated atherosclerosis occurs without elevated LDL-cholesterol and that the inhibitors of the vitamin K2–osteocalcin link, which are present in hydrogenated vegetable fats and oils, are important culprits in atherosclerosis and other lifestyle diseases. Like Professor Okuyama, I believe that the current harmful recommendations in lipid nutrition from WHO and other authoritative organizations are not acceptable and should be revised as soon as possible.

When drug industry-sponsored trials cannot be examined and questioned by independent researchers, science ceases to exist and becomes nothing more than marketing. Ignoring and misinterpreting the numerous studies which contradict the cholesterol hypothesis is a method which has been used by guideline authors for decades. There is strong evidence that high total or LDL-cholesterol is not the cause of atherosclerosis or cardiovascular disease.

The new guidelines conflict with evidence-based research, which clearly demonstrates that an elevated level of cholesterol is not a cause of heart disease. The persistence in focusing on LDL-cholesterol as the cause, and hence on the purported value of lowering LDL-cholesterol, continues to be counterproductive.

Sherif Sultan
Professor of Vascular and Endovascular Surgery
Chairman of the Western Vascular Institute
President of the International Society for Vascular Surgery
Galway, Ireland

Acknowledgments

We are very grateful to our English editor, Caryn Jones, of ThinkSCIENCE (Tokyo, Japan) for her support in publishing this manuscript.

1. How the Cholesterol Hypothesis Lost Credibility: A Brief Summary

Over the past several decades, the development of lipid nutrition has been intertwined with the cholesterol hypothesis, which states that increasing the polyunsaturated/saturated ratio of dietary lipids is effective in lowering blood cholesterol levels and thereby preventing atherosclerotic cardiovascular disease (ASCVD). Empirical equations clinically deduced in the 1960s by Keys et al. [1] and Hegsted et al. [2] were often used to predict the changes in plasma cholesterol levels as functions of the changes in dietary cholesterol, saturated fatty acids, and polyunsaturated fatty acids (PUFA), essentially linoleic acid (LA) from vegetable oils. Other equations have since been proposed, such as that by Derr et al. [3]: $\Delta TC = 2.3\Delta C14:0 + 3.0\Delta C16:0 - 0.8\Delta C18:0 - 1.0\Delta PUFA$, where Δ indicates the change by intervention. With this equation, saturated fatty acid with 18 carbons and no double bond (stearic acid; 18:0) was almost as effective as PUFA in lowering total cholesterol (TC) levels in young men. All of these equations were derived from interventions of around 1 month's duration. However, over the longer term, large-scale clinical trials aimed at lowering TC levels by dietary intervention demonstrated no significant decrease in TC levels after either 7 years of intervention (Multiple Risk Factor Intervention [MRFIT] Study, 1982) [4] or 10 years of intervention (Helsinki Businessmen Study, 1991) [5]. These findings are not necessarily surprising though, given that the MRFIT Study included stepped care treatments for hypertension and counseling for cigarette smoking, which are factors known not to affect plasma cholesterol levels significantly.

The cholesterol hypothesis was also the basis for the lipid nutritional recommendations made by a group of scientists from Harvard University School of Public Health (hereafter the Harvard U SPH group). The group reported that dietary saturated fatty acids and cholesterol, as well as the Keys score, were positively associated with age-adjusted myocardial infarction (MI) mortality, although the statistical significance of the correlation disappeared when adjusted for multivariate risk factors and further by fiber intake (Health Professionals Follow-up Study) [6]. Similarly, the multivariate relative risk of cardiovascular disease (CVD) was found not to be associated with cholesterol intake in the 14-year follow-up study [7]. Given these findings, it is difficult for us to understand how the Harvard U SPH group can recommend lipid nutrition based on the cholesterol hypothesis [8,9].

1.1. Lipid Nutrition Based on the Cholesterol Hypothesis Is Risky

The large-scale MRFIT Study was one of the trials expected to demonstrate the usefulness of controlling risk factors such as smoking, hypertension, and high TC levels by lifestyle intervention for the prevention of coronary heart disease (CHD) [4]. However, while smoking rate was significantly reduced, no significant reductions were noted in blood pressure, TC level, or mortality rates for CHD and all causes. Among the subgroup with hypertension and electrocardiographic anomaly, the CHD and all-cause mortality rates were actually higher in the intervention group, as we have pointed out previously [10]. In the Helsinki Businessmen Study [5], which involved longer-term dietary intervention, participants were followed for 15 years, including an initial 5-year period when they took hypotensive and cholesterol-lowering (non-statin) drugs. The CHD and all-cause mortality rates were found to be higher in the intervention group, and the difference in mortality rates widened between the control and intervention groups after several years, indicating that longer periods of follow-up are required in dietary intervention trials for clear differences in outcomes to become evident. No difference was noted in cholesterol levels at 10 years of intervention.

In the 28-year follow-up study of the Helsinki Businessmen Study [11], Strandberg et al. referred to their conclusions from the earlier 15-year follow-up study [5] differently. Reporting them now with three additional groups (the excluded group and refused group in the original study [5] and the low-risk group), they stated that the traditional risk factors of smoking, blood pressure, and cholesterol were associated with higher mortality. Adding these three subgroups is not a scientifically appropriate way to obtain these obviously different conclusions. Perhaps strong pressure from related industries and/or authoritative scholars was behind the modification of their initial conclusions. Nevertheless, industry-oriented scientists have made use of the latter conclusions, ignoring the earlier evidence that the intervention group had higher CVD and all-cause mortality rates.

Recently, using new statistical methods, Ramsden's group analyzed data recovered from two studies, the Diet Heart Study (2016) [12] and the Minnesota Coronary Experiment (1968–1973) [13]. Their reanalysis of the Diet Heart Study data found that both the CHD and all-cause mortality rates were significantly higher in the intervention group. In the Minnesota Coronary Experiment, they found no clinical benefit of the dietary intervention, which was based on the cholesterol hypothesis, although plasma TC levels were decreased significantly by the intervention [13].

The period of intervention is an important factor affecting plasma TC levels. For example, dietary changes in saturated fatty acids and PUFA affect plasma TC levels by a factor of 100% within 1 week [10], and the various equations cited above were obtained after about 1 month of intervention. Both the Diet Heart Study and the Minnesota Coronary Experiment revealed 14% lower TC levels in the intervention groups after ≥1 year of intervention, but no significant decrease in TC levels was observed after either 6 years in the MRFIT Study [4] or 10 years in the Helsinki Businessmen Study [5].

Needless to say, the findings of observational studies by the Harvard U SPH group provide working hypotheses that need to be proven by intervention trials. Such intervention trials have already been published [5,12,13], and enough evidence from randomized controlled trials (RCTs) has been published to convince us and many other scientists that the Harvard U SPH group's nutritional recommendations based on the cholesterol hypothesis are risky for the prevention of CHD and the reduction of all-cause deaths, as summarized above. In an early review in 1990, Muldoon reported no significant decrease in TC levels or CHD mortality had been observed, but that intervention groups had significantly increased rates of cancer mortality and violent deaths (deaths from accident, violence, trauma, and suicide) [14]. In a more recent 2015 meta-analysis [15], Harcombe revealed risk ratios (intervention vs. control) for all-cause mortality and CHD mortality of 0.996 (95% CI 0.865 to 1.147) and 0.989 (95% CI 0.784 to 1.247), respectively, from seven RCTs. Thus, it is more than clear that the intervention trials based on the cholesterol hypothesis afforded no benefits for the prevention of CHD and, in fact, could be risky by increasing violent deaths and cancer mortality [10,16].

The Finnish Mental Hospital Study [17] appears to be the only clinical trial that the Harvard U SPH group and their supporters depend on for their claim that increasing the PUFA/saturated fat ratio is useful for the prevention of CHD. However, there are critical defects in the design and conclusions of this study. We closely scrutinized the Finnish Mental Hospital Study and found that its findings are not in fact appropriate to support the mainstream lipid nutrition recommendations for the following four reasons.

1. This was a cross-over study (6 years in one hospital and 6 years in another), and it is likely that the first 6 years of dietary treatment carried over its nutritional effects to the next, as implied by the findings of the Helsinki Businessmen Study [5,11].
2. This was not an RCT as the physicians in charge were not blinded to which type of diet the participants were receiving. In such case, the most reliable endpoint is all-cause mortality, for which no difference was found between the two dietary groups.
3. This was not a controlled study; the amount of sugar varied by almost 50% between the diet periods.
4. Systolic (SBP) and diastolic (DBP) blood pressure at one of the hospitals was higher in the control group than in the intervention group (mean SBP, 148 vs. 140, respectively; percent SBP $\geq$160, 28.6% vs. 19.2%; mean DBP, 94 vs. 87; and percent DBP $\geq$95, 49.7% vs. 21.5%). In particular, the odds ratio of patients with DBP $\geq$95 in the control group vs the intervention group was estimated at

3.6 (95% confidence interval 2.3, 5.6; $p < 0.0000001$), although the authors did not show the data used in the statistical analysis.

Moreover, in the other hospital where blood pressure values were not so different, the control group's use of both phenothiazines and psychostimulants, both of which are cardiotoxic, was more than double the intervention group's. These differences could have substantially contributed to the difference in cardiovascular events found.

The Finnish Mental Hospital Study [17] has often been cited in support of the Harvard U SPH group's hypotheses, but mostly by industry-oriented people who do not recognize the criticism of the study's conclusions [18,19]. As we clearly see it, the study cannot provide adequate support for the mainstream recommendations that increasing the PUFA/saturated fat ratio in the diet is beneficial for the prevention of CHD.

1.2. Pharmacological Mechanisms of Excess Linoleic Acid and Relative n-3 Deficiency Syndrome

As the cholesterol hypothesis became widely and mistakenly accepted in nutrition science, we looked at ways to highlight the problem. We decided to compare the effects of linoleic-rich safflower oil and α-linolenic-rich perilla (seed) oil in various animal models. These two vegetable oils are suitable for comparing LA (n-6) and α-linolenic acid (ALA, n-3) because, while they have similar proportions of saturated and monounsaturated fatty acids, their proportions of LA and ALA constitute a major difference between them. Neither oil exhibited activity that induced stroke or shortened survival, activity that was found later in stroke-prone spontaneously hypertensive (SHRSP) rats [20,21]. As summarized in Table 1, we found that compared with safflower oil, perilla oil suppressed carcinogenesis and metastasis, suppressed the production of allergic lipid mediators and platelet-activating factor (PAF), suppressed antigen-induced anaphylaxis and platelet aggregability, and improved learning and memory behavior in the second generation of rats.

After Dyerberg et al. reported different disease patterns between native Greenland and mainland Danish populations in 1978 [22], research started on changing the n-6/n-3 balance of diets. It was found that the effects of changing this balance were similar to those shown by fish oil supplementation in regular diets. There were clear merits to using animal models to examine changes in the n-6/n-3 balance of different vegetable oil diets. One was that it made chronic dietary manipulation possible, for example, through generations. Another was that the diet containing 10 wt.% perilla oil exhibited prophylactic activity toward allergic and inflammatory diseases including carcinogenesis, without noticeable adverse effects on animal physiology such as teratogenicity and growth in the second generation of some strains of rats, as compared with the diet containing safflower oil (Table 1).

Table 1. Nutritional effects of long-term feeding of perilla (seed) oil with a n-6/n-3 ratio of 15/65 (percent of total fatty acids) and safflower oil with a ratio of 78/1.

Reference	Experimental Models	Effects of Perilla Oil vs. Safflower Oil
Yamamoto et al., *J Lipid Res* **1987**, *28*, 144–151.	Learning ability evaluated by the brightness-darkness discrimination test in rats	Learning and memory ability of the rats through two generations was better in the rats fed the perilla oil diet
Hori et al., *Chem Pharm Bull* **1987**, *35*, 3925–3927.	Pulmonary metastasis of intravenously injected Yoshida sarcoma in Donryu rats	Number of metastatic foci in the lung was smaller in the rats fed the perilla oil diet
Hashimoto et al., *Prostaglandins* **1988**, *3*, 3–16.	Release of leukotrienes from rat peritoneal leukocytes stimulated with calcium ionophore	Production of leukotrienes derived from arachidonic acid was suppressed in the rats fed the perilla oil diet
Watanabe et al., *Chem Pharm Bull* **1989**, *37*, 1572–1575.	Collagen-induced platelet aggregation using rat platelet-rich plasma	Aggregability of rat platelets was lower in the rats fed the perilla oil diet
Hirose et al., *Carcinogenesis* **1990**, *11*, 731–735.	Mammary gland and colon carcinogenesis induced by sequential administration of DMBA and dimethylhydrazine in SD rats	Colon tumor incidence was significantly lower in the rats fed the perilla oil diet
Narisawa et al., *Cancer* **1994**, *73*, 2069–2075.	N-methyl-N-nitrosourea-induced colon carcinogenesis in SD rats	Incidence of colon carcinogenesis was significantly lower in the mice fed the perilla oil diet
Watanabe et al., *J Nutr* **1994**, *124*, 1566–1573.	Antigen-induced anaphylactic shock in mice	Mortality rate of anaphylactic death was lower in the mice fed the perilla oil diet
Okaniwa et al., *Biol Pharm Bull* **1996**, *19*, 536–540.	Effect of shifting the diets at weaning	Inferior learning behavior of rats fed a safflower oil diet was reversed by shifting to a perilla oil diet at weaning
Matsuba S, Itoh M, Joh T, et al. *Prostaglandins Leukot Essent Fatty Acids* **1998**, *59*, 317–323.	Effect of dietary linoleate/alpha-linolenate balance on experimentally induced gastric injury	Lowering n-6/n-3 ratio is safe in a gastric ulcer model of the rat

Abbreviations: DMBA, 2,4-dimethoxybenzaldehyde; PAF, platelet-activating factor; SD, Sprague Dawley; SHRSP, stroke-prone spontaneously hypertensive.

The n-6/n-3 ratios of dietary lipids are reflected in tissue lipids, particularly in membrane phospholipid fractions. The phospholipid fatty acid compositions are kept within a certain range by specific acyltransferases and phospholipases [23–25] but are variable depending on changes in the n-6/n-3 ratios of diets. In the brain and retina, mainly it is the ARA/DHA ratio that varies, while in the liver and kidney the ARA/(EPA+DHA) ratio varies. These fatty acids are incorporated into membrane phospholipid tissue specifically and are phospholipid class specific. The size of the seats occupied by these n-6 and n-3 fatty acids in the membrane phospholipids also appears to be restricted to a certain range, and the fatty acids compete with each other to take the seats. For example, analysis of blood samples from US adults (n = 1015) [26] revealed that increasing n-3 fatty acids (EPA, DPA, DHA) was clearly associated with decreasing ARA (n-6) in blood lipids, as in vitro enzyme assays roughly predicted (Figure 1). Although the major n-6 fatty acid in our diet is LA (n-6), of which about 10 g is ingested per day, decreasing LA intake is not very effective in reducing the proportion of ARA (n-6) in mammals. It is an essential fatty acid and there appear to be mechanisms to maintain tissue LA within a certain range. The enzymes incorporating LA and ARA into lipids are different, and both EPA (n-3) and DHA (n-3) can compete effectively with ARA (n-6) to occupy the seats in membrane lipids [10].

1.3. Pharmacological Implications of the n-6/n-3 Balance of Dietary and Tissue Lipids

After being released from phospholipids by phospholipase A2 and lipases, PUFA with 20 carbons and ≥3 double bonds (HUFA) are converted to prostaglandins (PG), thromboxanes (TX), leukotrienes (LT), and several other eicosanoids with different physiological activities (Figure 2). ARA is converted to thrombotic TX A2 in platelets and to anti-thrombotic PG I2 in the endothelial cells of blood vessels; EPA is converted to TX A3 and PG I3, but to a lesser extent compared with TX A2 and PG I2. Similarly, LT B5 produced from EPA through the 5-lipoxygenase pathway in neutrophils and monocytes exhibits much lower chemoattractant activity than LT B4 produced from arachidonic acid (ARA) [31,32]. This is the basis for recommending lowering the tissue ARA/EPA ratio by dietary means for the prevention of thrombotic diseases and allergic, inflammatory diseases including carcinogenesis and atherogenesis.

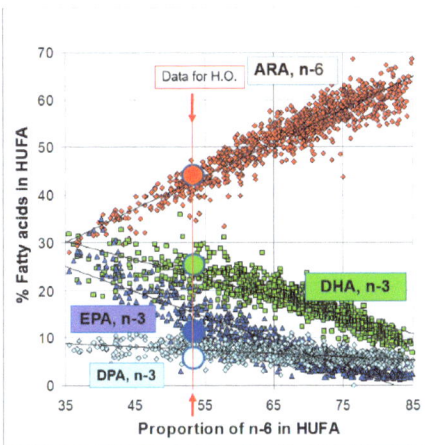

Figure 1. Balance of competing n-6 and n-3 highly unsaturated fatty acids (HUFA) in tissue lipids, as obtained in an analysis of fatty acids in blood samples from 1015 US adults [26]. HUFA have ≥20 carbon chains and ≥3 double bonds, and competition between n-6 HUFA and n-3 HUFA has been clearly demonstrated [26,27]. Figure is reproduced with permission from Ref. [26,28]. Overlaid on the dataset are the HUFA compositions of blood lipids of one of the Japanese authors (H.O.), plotted in large circles. H.O.'s n-6/n-3 ratios were much smaller than those for most of the American participants. Lands [29] pioneered research into the relationship between dietary fatty acids and diseases, and Smith et al. [30] clarified the molecular mechanisms that convert n-6 and n-3 fatty acids to eicosanoids through cyclooxygenases and lipoxygenases.

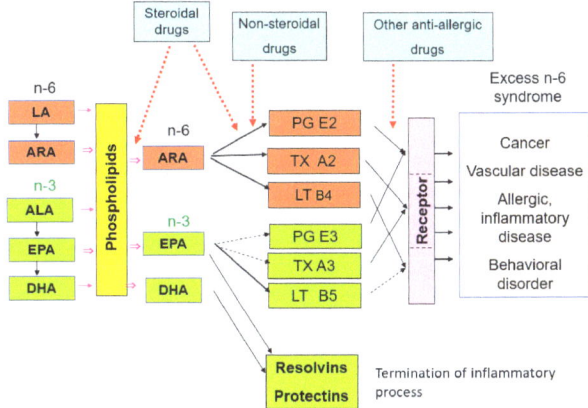

Figure 2. A simplified schematic of the relationships among enzymes incorporating n-6 and n-3 fatty acids into phospholipids, the conversion to eicosanoids, inhibitors of the metabolism, and their consequences. See the text for details.

Another group of eicosanoids, namely, LT C, LT D, and LT E, are named peptide LT as they include the glutathione (GSH) molecule and/or its metabolites. These are mainly produced in white blood cells (mast cells and eosinophils). LT C4 (formerly called SRS-A) exhibits bronchoconstriction activity. Whereas the bronchoconstrictive activity of histamine derived from histidine on smooth muscle cells is relatively transient, that of LT C4 is longer lasting, as in the case of asthma. In blood vessels, LT C4 relaxes smooth muscle and increases capillary permeability, thereby increasing inflammation. Thus, LT C4 serves to initiate inflammatory processes, and its persistency is a serious problem. Accordingly, various inhibitors of this ARA-eicosanoid cascade have been developed, and more than 90% of the anti-allergic drugs registered in Japan exert activity to inhibit this cascade.

EPA is also a substrate for the biosynthesis of corresponding peptide LTs such as LT C5, LT D5, and LT E5. Although conflicting results have been reported for the relative potencies of LTs derived from ARA and EPA using in vitro bioassays, the potencies of LT C5 and LT D5 to induce gastric vascular damage are much lower than those of LT C4 and LT D4 from ARA in rats. These differences in the activity of eicosanoids derived from ARA and EPA are the basis for recommending lowering the tissue ARA/EPA ratio by dietary manipulation [10]. It is important to note that the physiological activity reported for these peptide LTs differs considerably among publications [33–35].

In animal experiments comparing linoleic-rich safflower oil and α-linoleic-rich perilla oil, feeding these oils through two generations consistently resulted in significant differences in behavior that are associated with an altered ARA/DHA ratio [36]. In aged rats, learning and memory performance was superior and average survival time was longer by 10% in the perilla oil group [20], but in mice, locomotor activity was similar between the two groups. These findings became the basis for the so-called anti-aging activity of perilla oil (Table 1, p. 5). More importantly, in rats, the inferior learning ability induced by n-3 deficiency in the safflower oil group was restored by feeding perilla oil after weaning [37], which led to clinical trials comparing the behavioral performance of newborn babies with or without fish oil-supplemented milk [38].

In a case-control study conducted in China, Hamazaki's group [39] found an inverse association of suicide attempts with erythrocyte ARAn-6 levels, and this paved the way to clinical studies on dietary n-6 and n-3 fatty acids and human behavior. This link between dietary n-6 and n-3 fatty acids and human behavior is one of the major research topics of the Japan Society for Lipid Nutrition. Also, Hibbeln's group [40] in the US has examined the impact of these fatty acids on human psychiatric performance clinically.

With animal experiments on dietary n-6 and n-3 fatty acids as a starting point, many clinical results have now been published. These results, obtained in part from the studies cited above, indicate lipid nutrition is closely correlated with neuronal, psychiatric, and behavioral performance. As we mentioned in a recent publication, we have correlated the rapidly decreasing birth rate in Japan with increased intake of some types of vegetable oils that affect mental aspects of behavior as well as physiological aspects [28].

1.4. Essential Roles of the Arachidonic Acid Cascade

LA is essential to the ARA cascade and thus to the maintenance of proper growth, reproductive physiology, and skin health. However, over- and unbalanced production of eicosanoids from ARA can cause persistent inflammation leading to pathological conditions [41]. The essential amount of LA for humans is 0.5%–1% of energy, and on average people ingest approximately 3% of energy from food materials such as grains, animal foods, and plant foods. Currently, authoritative organizations recommend doubling the amount of LA in foods; the American Heart Association (AHA) recommends 12% of energy in the form of LA, while a Japanese government agency gives no upper limit of LA intake, after withdrawing the upper limit (10% of energy) in 2015 without giving a clear explanation for setting a new target (Overview of Dietary Reference Intakes for Japanese (2015), Ministry of Health, Labour and Welfare Japan.[1]

The ranges of dietary LA n-6/ALA n-3 ratios and tissue ARA/EPA ratios need to be carefully estimated in different tissues where prostaglandin E2 (PGE2) plays important roles as a pathological mediator or protective mediator. In a water-immersion, stress-induced ulcer model, the dietary n-6/n-3 ratio can be lowered by roughly 1/1 or even lower [42], a level which is difficult to achieve by increasing intake of n-3 fatty acids under normal dietary conditions, as average intake of LA n-6 is ≥15 g/day in Japan (Figure 3, p. 10).

1.5. Anti-Inflammatory Hydroxylated Mediators Produced from EPA and DHA

The anti-inflammatory activity of n-3 fatty acids, particularly EPA and DHA, has been explained in terms of eicosanoid balance and competitive aspects of n-6 and n-3 fatty acids in phospholipid metabolism [10,29]. Because eicosanoids function as local hormones, their plasma levels do not simply reflect the pathology of tissues, which makes the study of causal relationships rather complicated.

---

[1] See https://www.mhlw.go.jp/file/06-Seisakujouhou-10900000-Kenkoukyoku/Overview.pdf (accessed on 28 September 2020).

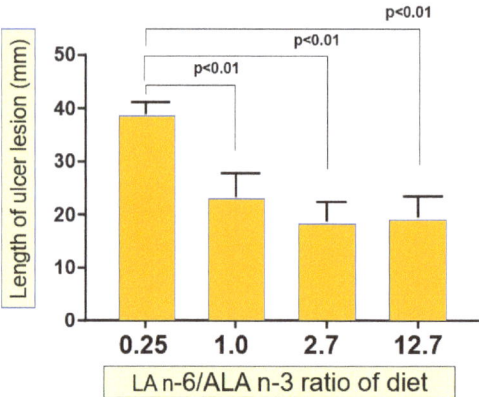

Figure 3. Effect of dietary n-6/n-3 ratio of dietary oils in a water-immersion, stress-induced gastric injury model. Rats were fed diets with different n-6/n-3 ratios by varying perilla oil and safflower oil as well as their mixtures. Water-immersion stress was loaded for 6 h and then the ulcer lesion was examined 24 h later [42]. Each column and bar represent the mean and SEM of 6 to 8 rats in each group. See the text for details. Figure is based on data from Ref. [42].

Another group of lipid mediator includes resolvins and protectins, hydroxyl or epoxy derivatives from EPA and DHA [43]. These lipid mediators are thought to serve to terminate inflammatory reactions caused by ARA metabolites [44,45]. Hundreds of hydroxyl and epoxy fatty acids have been identified by instrumental analysis, but their pharmacological activity has been determined only in part. Nevertheless, ARA, EPA, and DHA are known to be involved in the initiation and termination of inflammation, and it has been clinically proven that lowering the n-6/n-3 ratio of dietary lipids is effective in the prevention of atherogenesis, carcinogenesis, and aging processes [10,29,46]. Other n-6 and n-3 fatty acids are also metabolized to hydroxy or epoxy derivatives.

Aside from the anti-inflammatory activity of n-3 fatty acids, we should also consider adverse effects of n-3 fatty acid intake from seafood. Findings reported for Danish populations suggest that excessive intake of EPA and DHA augments the onset of cerebral hemorrhage (apoplexy). Mortality from apoplexy was found to be 1.7-fold higher in a native Greenland population than in a mainland Danish population [47]. Fish oil n-3 fatty acids are effective in suppressing platelet aggregability, and in fact a bleeding tendency was noted in the native Greenland population [22]. However, the summary from the working group of the International Society for Studies on Fatty Acids and Lipids (ISSFAL) stated that clinical studies on fish oil supplementation failed to demonstrate an increased bleeding tendency as an adverse effect [48].

We now interpret these studies' findings as a potential shortage of vitamin K2 (VK2) among the Native Greenland population, given that seafood in general is not rich in VK2 (Figure 4). VK is detectable only in sea urchin and abalone, not in the 130 other kinds of seafood (including whale) in the 2015 Standard Tables of Food Composition in Japan.[2] Given that more precise data on VK in seafood (including seal) is still needed, it is interesting to know the status of the VK2–osteocalcin link in people who depend mostly on a diet of seafood.

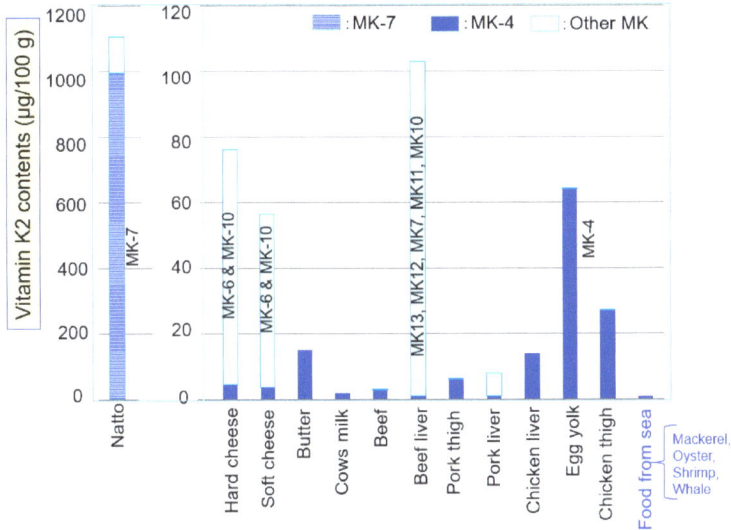

Figure 4. Vitamin K2 contents of common foods. Data from Refs. [49] and [50]. Seafood included in "Food from sea" does not contain Vitamin K1 as well. Figure is based on data from Refs. [49,50].

1.6. Platelet-Activating Factor and Ethanol Amide of Fatty Acids (Anandamide)

PAF is a phospholipid mediator with a structure of 1-alkylether, 2-acetyl-glycerol 3-phosphocholine [51]. In injured tissues, it activates platelet aggregation for hemostasis at very low concentrations (10^{-12} mol/L). It is also produced in neutrophils, eosinophils, monocytes/macrophages, and vascular endothelial cells and serves as a mediator of inflammation, anaphylaxis, and bronchoconstriction. In the case of bacterial infection, endotoxin induces PAF production, leading to hypotension, decreased blood flow to the heart, and eventually shock.

In PAF precursor molecules in membranes, the 2-position is enriched with ARA and EPA depending on the dietary n-6/n-3 balance, and ARA and EPA are released upon stimulation with phospholipase A2 and/or CoA-independent transacylase to

---

[2] See https://www.mext.go.jp/en/policy/science_technology/policy/title01/detail01/1374030.htm (accessed on 28 September 2020).

form lyso-PAF (Figure 5). In rats fed ALA-rich perilla oil, the production of PAF from stimulated leukocytes was 50% less than that in rats fed LA-rich safflower oil [52], which reflected a 30% decrease in CoA-independent transacylase and/or phospholipase A2 activity [53]. Thus, the production of PAF can be regulated safely by perilla oil, but EPA is not effective because it is released equally to ARA from the precursor 1-alkenyl-2-acyl-glycerophospholipids. In our experience, this was the only case in which ALA(n-3) was more effective than EPA(n-3) in suppressing ARA-related lipid metabolism. Natural PAF antagonists have also been found in plants, but their applicability in regulating platelet aggregation and preventing CHD appears to require more time.

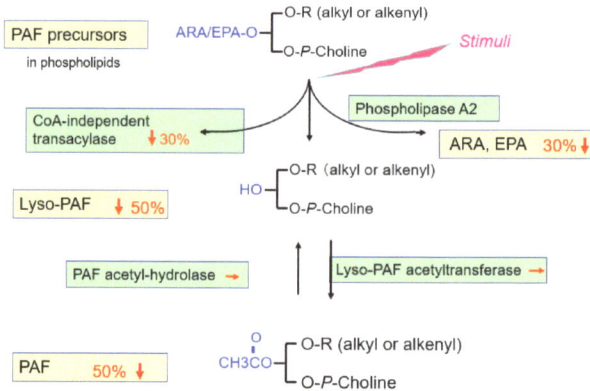

Figure 5. Dietary high-ALA perilla oil suppresses PAF production in rat leukocytes compared with high-LA safflower oil. Figure is based on data from Refs. [52,53]. See the text for details. *P*, phosphate; PAF, platelet activating factor.

Another physiologically active fatty acid derivative is anandamide. An active component of the cannabis plant is tetrahydrocannabinol (THC), which binds to receptors (CB1 and CB2) expressed in the central and peripheral nerves. The endogenous agonists for these receptors are arachidonoyl-ethanolamide and 2-arachidonoyl-glycerol [54–56]. The molecules containing ARA (n-6) are more potent than derivatives containing EPA (n-3) or other fatty acids. Reducing the dietary n-6/n-3 ratio results in reducing ARA-containing endocannabinoids. This endocannabinoid system is reported to be involved in numerous physiological and cognitive processes, including fertility, pregnancy, pre- and postnatal development, appetite, pain sensation, mood, and memory. Oleoyl amide (oleic acid ethanol amide), which is found in cerebrospinal fluid, may be involved in sleep. It would seem, then, that this group of fatty acid ethanol amides has much to do with the topics of this review on dietary lipids that affect physical and mental activity and their disorders.

1.7. Gene Technology Applied to Lipid Nutrition

The usefulness of reducing the n-6/n-3 ratio of dietary and tissue lipids for the prevention of inflammatory diseases has been proven from the perspectives of nutrition (Table 1, Figures 1–3), pharmacology in terms of the action mechanisms of steroidal and non-steroidal anti-inflammatory drugs, and gene technology. The latter includes gene-knockout models involved in the ARA cascade, and a transgenic mouse model expressing the *C. elegans fat-1* gene encoding an n-3 fatty acid desaturase. These *fat-1* transgenic mice can produce n-3 fatty acids from dietary and tissue linoleic acid (n-6) [57], leading to abundant n-3 fatty acids with reduced levels of n-6 fatty acids in their tissues. Feeding an identical diet (high in n-6) to the transgenic mice and wildtype littermates can produce a different n-6/n-3 balance (e.g., ARA/EPA ratio) in membrane phospholipids. This model exhibits resistance to inflammation (inflammatory bowel disease, acute hepatitis, retinal degeneration disease, pancreatitis, acute pulmonary disorders, diabetes, atherosclerosis, and asthma) and carcinogenesis (melanoma and colorectal, prostatic, and hepatic cancers). The model is also being used to clarify the requirement of n-3 fatty acids for hippocampal neurogenesis in depression [58].

1.8. Why Some Clinical Studies Have Failed to Show the Effectiveness of n-3 Lipids in Suppressing Allergic and Inflammatory Diseases

In animal models, dietary modifications to lower the tissue ARA/(EPA+DHA) ratio are effective in suppressing allergic, inflammatory diseases related to carcinogenesis, atherogenesis, and allergic hyperreactivity, which is consistent with the results from clinical observational studies [10]. However, a recent Cochrane database systematic review suggests that increasing EPA and DHA has little or no beneficial effect on mortality or cardiovascular health [59], and that increasing ALA may slightly reduce the number of CVD events, CHD mortality, and arrhythmia. However, as we have discussed already, RCT trials have not been performed because of the cost-performance problems associated with evaluating the effectiveness of n-3 lipids in suppressing allergic and inflammatory diseases. No priority has been given to evaluating food constituents such as EPA and DHA, so we must draw conclusions from observational studies. The results of the Seven Countries study and the French, Indian, and Okinawan paradoxes can be explained in terms of difference in seafood intake [10,29]. Moreover, the findings of an epidemiological study on CVD in a fishing and farming village in Chiba Prefecture, Japan, prompted mechanistic studies to be conducted using >95% pure ethyl ester of EPA: as early as the 1980s, clinical trials in Japan demonstrated that EPA suppressed platelet aggregability, lowered blood viscosity, increased PGI2-like substance, and increased red blood cell deformability [60–64]. So, why then have some clinical studies failed to show such effectiveness? Let's look at a few examples.

Since 1961, the Hisayama Study, a population-based prospective cohort study designed to evaluate risk factors for lifestyle-related diseases in a general Japanese population, has been conducting prospective follow-up surveys with participants aged ≥40 years [65]. Positive correlations were reported between blood EPA level, inflammatory markers, and CVD morbidity. The participants (n = 3103, aged ≥40 years) were followed for 5.1 years. In the group with high-sensitivity C-reactive protein (HS-CRP) levels of ≥1.0 mg/L, the serum EPA/ARA ratio (quartile) was inversely associated with CHD events (hazard ratio [HR] 2.23, p for trend = 0.007), but the group with HS-CRP <1.0 mg/L showed no significant associations. In the case of stroke, no associations were observed for the DHA/AA ratio. The results are consistent with the presumed mechanism of atherosclerosis, in which persistent inflammation following microbial infection is an early event. A weakness of the Hisayama Study though is the insufficient number of cases (127 cases) to perform an accurate analysis.

Discrepancies over the effectiveness of n-3 fatty acids for the prevention of CVD and other inflammatory diseases are likely attributable to differences in the extent to which the phospholipid ARA/EPA ratio is modified (Figure 1, p. 7). In a longitudinal study using intima-media thickness (IMT) as a marker of atherosclerosis, IMT was found to be lowest in Japanese Americans living in Hawaii, followed by Caucasian Americans living in the mainland USA and then Japanese living in Japan [66] (Figure 6). IMT was inversely associated with marine n-3 fatty acids in plasma lipids ($p < 0.004$) in Japanese living in Japan, who had EPA levels exceeding 6% of the total, but not in Americans with much lower EPA levels. Marine n-3 fatty acids must account for a significant proportion of plasma lipids in order to lower the ARA/EPA ratios of tissue lipids and CVD mortality (Figure 1). Interestingly, IMT differed greatly between the Japanese Americans living in Hawaii and Japanese living in Japan who had the same n-3 levels (at about 6%). This indicates that factors other than plasma n-3 fatty acids are involved in atherosclerosis, such as vegetable fats and oils, as we discuss next.

We suspect that the Cochrane database systematic review covered populations with relatively small changes in tissue ARA/EPA ratios and relatively short periods of intervention. Lipid nutrition guidelines should emphasize the importance of the extent of modifications to tissue lipids [10,29] and the period of intervention should be long enough for the effects of EPA and DHA to be exerted [5].

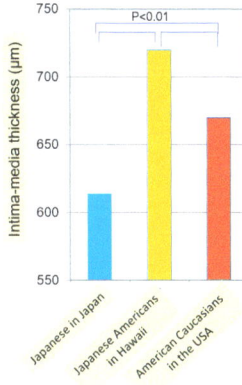 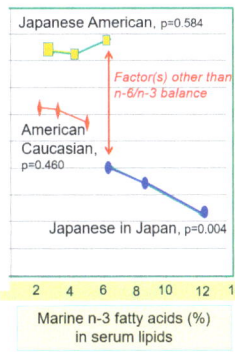

Figure 6. Comparison of atherosclerosis markers among Japanese living in Japan, Japanese Americans living in Hawaii, and American Caucasians living in the mainland USA, as revealed by the ERA-JUMP study [66]. Among the three groups, intima-media thickness was proportional to coronary calcification (%) (data not shown). Figure is based on data from Ref. [66].

1.9. Critical Evaluation of the American Heart Association's Basis for Recommending Increased Intake of Vegetable Oils Instead of Animal Fats

The AHA's presidential advisory on dietary fats and CVD consists of the following [67].

1. RCTs that lowered intake of dietary saturated fat and replaced it with polyunsaturated vegetable oil reduced CVD by around 30%, similar to the reduction achieved by statin treatment.
2. Prospective observational studies in many populations showed that lower intake of saturated fat coupled with higher intake of polyunsaturated and monounsaturated fat is associated with lower rates of CVD and of other major causes of death and all-cause mortality.
3. Replacing saturated fats with unsaturated fats lowers low-density lipoprotein cholesterol, a cause of atherosclerosis, linking biological evidence with the incidence of CVD in populations and in clinical trials.

Based on these key elements, the AHA strongly concluded that lowering intake of saturated fat and replacing it with unsaturated fats, especially polyunsaturated fats, will lower the incidence of CVD. The 2015-2020 Dietary Guidelines for Americans follow this advisory.

The AHA presidential advisory cited the Finnish Mental Hospital Study [17] as important evidence. However, as we described earlier in this chapter, our critical evaluation of the study highlighted four reasons why it is not a reliable RCT. Moreover, we do not accept the interpretation that high low-density lipoprotein cholesterol (LDL-C) is causative for CVD and that statins are effective for lowering CVD. We have previously argued that high levels of LDL-C serve as a predictor of longevity and also that RCTs performed after 2004–2005 (when new regulations on clinical trials came to effect) failed to demonstrate that statins decrease objective measures of CVD, such as MI mortality and/or all-cause mortality [10–19]. Furthermore, clinical observations support the data on the pharmacological mechanisms of statins that they actually accelerate atherosclerosis and heart failure [68,69]. To support the AHA presidential advisory, scientists would need not only to disregard the published findings on the adverse effects of some types of vegetable fats and oils, but also disregard the evidence we have presented so far in this review. In fact, Teicholz and Thorn [18] classified opinion leaders involved in the AHA presidential advisory into those who accept the advisory but have conflict of interest (COI) problems and those who do not accept the advisory and have no COI problems. Currently, two inconsistent recommendations are put forward in lipid nutrition for the prevention of CVD, one by industry-oriented people and the other by those emphasizing the mechanism-based perspective. The production and consumption of oilseeds, such as rapeseed, soybean, corn, olive, and many others, are now of serious concern in many countries and regions of the world.

We want to end this chapter with a critical evaluation of the Prospective Urban Rural Study, known as the PURE Study [70]. In this large-scale study, individuals aged 35–70 years (enrolled during 2003 and 2013) in 18 countries from five continents were followed for a median 7.4 years. Dietary intake of 135,335 individuals was recorded, and the association of estimated percentage energy from nutrients with total mortality and major cardiovascular disease (fatal cardiovascular disease + myocardial infarction + stroke + heart failure) was examined. Adjustments were made for age, sex, education, waist-to-hip ratio, smoking, physical activity, diabetes, urban or rural location, center, geographic region, and energy intake. The three major conclusions that Dehghan et al. reported for the study were as follows [70].

1. Carbohydrate intake was associated with an increased risk of total mortality but not with the risk of CVD mortality.
2. Intake of total fat and each type of fat was associated with lower risk of total mortality (total fat: HR 0.77, $p < 0.0001$; saturated fat, HR 0.86, $p = 0.0088$; monounsaturated fat: HR 0.81, $p < 0.0001$; and polyunsaturated fat: HR 0.80, $p < 0.0001$).
3. Higher saturated fat intake was associated with lower risk of stroke (HR 0.79, $p = 0.0498$).

There are, however, problems with the PURE study.

1. The results from this large-scale observational study do not support the Harvard U SPH group's recommendations nor our own, and we urge caution in the interpretation of its results because there are critical problems associated with its planning and methods. Detailed data on nutrient intake is not readily available in all of the countries included, such as Argentina, Brazil, Canada, Chili, China, Columbia, India, Iran, Malaysia, Palestine Autonomous Region, and Pakistan.
2. The term "Polyunsaturates" appears not to include ingested vegetable oils (Methods section), and there are also no data given for the n-6/n-3 balance of PUFA.
3. The correlations shown between carbohydrates and disease incidence were not adjusted for the intake of other nutrients. For example, the subgroup with very high carbohydrate intake may have had low protein intake rather than excessive carbohydrate intake [71].
4. The Japanese population's experience during the period of polyunsaturated fats intake was 2.8 energy percent in 1960 (15 years after the end of the Second World War when people were living under relatively stable nutritional conditions) and 5.8 energy percent in 2010. In other words, Japanese people had no experience of intake outside this range. However, it is from outside this range that the authors of the PURE Study drew important conclusions [70].

So, despite this being one of the largest-scale observational studies reported to date, the applicability of the conclusions to the Japanese population are extremely limited and the recommendations are very likely to be wrong.

Chapter 1 Summary

Lipid nutrition based on the cholesterol hypothesis has lost its foundation and clinical trials based on the hypothesis have shown it to be harmful. In spite of the scientific evidence available, the so-called authoritative organizations that often have strong relationships with the food and drug industry still repeatedly recommend increasing the intake of PUFA from vegetable oils. Both n-6 and n-3 PUFA are converted to various physiologically active derivatives essential for the maintenance of physical and mental activity. In the current food environment, however, the balance of n-6 and n-3 fatty acids is too much in favor of n-6, and therefore lowering the n-6/n-3 ratio is recommended for the prevention of allergic and inflammatory diseases including ASCVD and cancer.

2. All Mainstream Guidelines in Lipid Nutrition Disregard Evidence That Some Types of Vegetable Fats and Oils Induce Stroke and Disrupt Endocrines

2.1. Toxicity of Some Types of Vegetable Fats and Oils Observed in Stroke-Prone Spontaneously Hypertensive Rats

Rapeseed oil contains two anti-nutritional factors, erucic acid (22:1n-9) that causes lipidosis in the heart and thyrotoxic glucosinolates that exhibit thyrotoxicity in rodents. Armed with this knowledge, scientists selected a variety of rapeseed with much lower levels of both factors and in 1974 created a double-low oil that they named canola oil. In the original rapeseed oil, more than half of the total fatty acids comprised erucic acid; however, in canola oils, erucic acid is currently <1% of the total and oleic acid accounts for >60% of the total. Because the linoleic acid content is relatively low (21%–32%) and α-linolenic acid content is high (9%–15%) compared with common vegetable oils, canola is recommended by many nutritionists as a cooking oil due to its relatively low n-6/n-3 ratio. (Figure S1 shows the fatty acid composition of some common fats and oils.)

Given that lipophilic substances are transferred easily to the brain, affecting behavior, and through the umbilical cord to fetal tissue, nutritional evaluation of fats and oils should be made by feeding test oils through two or more generations. This simple notion led one of our group (H.O.) to start feeding experiments with SHRSP rats, a strain established by Okamoto and Aoki in 1963 from conventional WKY/Kyoto rats by brother-sister mating of those exhibiting higher blood pressure [72–74].

Canola oil and evening primrose oil shortened survival by 40%, compared with fish oil and perilla (seed) oil (Figure 7, p. 20). The difference between high-linoleic soybean oil and perilla oil was about 10%. Even with the SHRSP rat strain, it took >500 days to complete a set of experiments. When 1% NaCl solution was loaded as drinking water, the difference in survival time between soybean oil and canola oil was roughly reproduced within <250 days. It should be noted that animals drink water when ingesting salty foods, but this model provides salt solution only; most of the experiments to simply compare survival times were performed under 1% NaCl loading unless otherwise stated. Different types of canola oil, traditional erucic acid-rich rapeseed oil, and various manufacturers' products were similarly toxic to SHRSP rats. Today, we now know that double-low rapeseed oils produced in different countries exhibit similar toxicity.

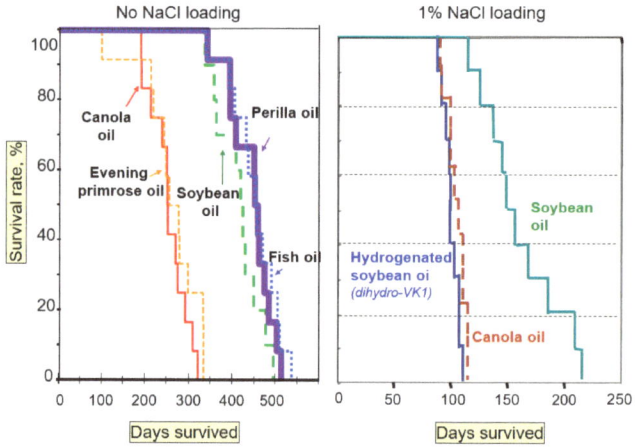

Figure 7. Survival of SHRSP male rats fed a diet containing 10 wt.% fat or oil from weaning at 4 weeks of age. Hydrogenation of soybean oil produced toxic substance(s) [75]. See the text for details. Figure 7 is reproduced with permission from Ref. [28].

In our first report on canola oil in 1996 [75], we reported that a mixture containing soybean oil/canola oil (3/1) significantly shortened survival in a dose-dependent manner; hence the tolerable daily intake (TDI) must be <6% of energy. We emphasize this point here because a Japanese administrative agency subsequently undervalued our report[3] describing the lack of data on the dose-dependent effects. We accept the criticism that larger numbers of animals and groups are required to obtain more accurate TDI values.

Following our request for collaboration to investigate the issue with canola oil, in 2000, Ratnayake's group at Health Canada [76,77] reported that olive oil and corn oil exhibited survival-shortening activity as well, and they proposed phytosterol as an anti-nutritional substance, even though olive oil contained the least amount of phytosterol (Figure 8). It was about this time when a specific-pathogen free colony of the SHRSP rat became available and we noticed significant differences in their sensitivity to canola oil toxicity. Each laboratory tends to maintain its colonies by mating the rats with high blood pressure. Currently, the SHRSP rat colony with a high sensitivity to canola toxicity is commercially available as SHRSP/*izm*.

---

[3] See the report by Nagata J, Health and Labor Sciences Research Grant 200500122A; https://mhlw-grants.niph.go.jp/niph/search/NISR00.do (accessed on 28 September 2020).

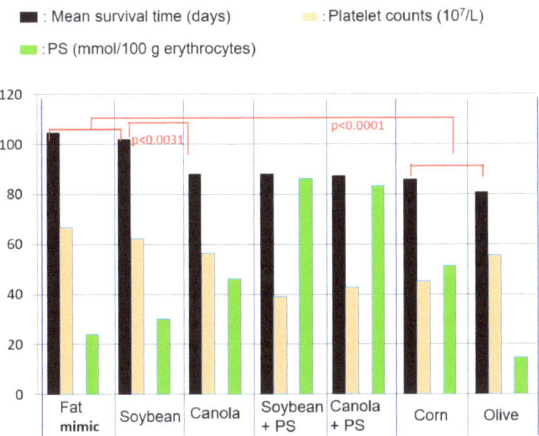

Figure 8. Effect of dietary olive oil, canola oil, and PS on the survival of SHRSP rats. Figure is based on data from Refs. [76,77]. Although PS shortened survival, it took 3-fold more PS to reproduce the toxicity of canola [78], and olive oil contained least amount of PS among the oils examined. PS, phytosterol; fat mimic, a mixture of vegetable oils and animal fats prepared to mimic the fatty acid composition ingested by the average Canadian.

A two-generation study found that dams' milk and pre-weaning diet affected the survival of the second-generation rats (Figure 9).

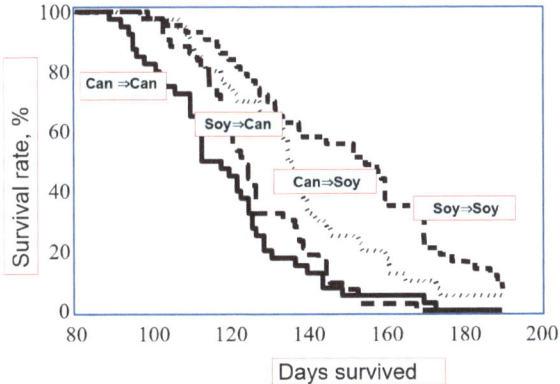

Figure 9. Dietary oil intake of dams affects the survival of offspring. SHRSP rats fed either canola oil diet (Can) or soybean oil diet (Soy) from 4 weeks of age were mated at 12 weeks of age (F0), and half of the offspring (F1) were weaned to the same diet as the dams' and the other half were weaned to a different diet. Male offspring raised under the same dietary conditions were pooled from four separate experiments and the results were statistically analyzed [79]. Figure is reproduced with permission from Ref. [28], with slight modifications.

2.2. Mechanisms of Canola Oil and Hydrogenated Oil Causing Toxicity

In male SHRSP rats fed canola oil or hydrogenated soybean oil, second-generation animals in the canola group had stroke, kidney injury, decreased platelet count, decreased testosterone levels in the testes, accelerated onset of diabetes, ectopic bone morphogenesis, and behavioral change compared with second-generation animals in the soybean group (see Table 1, , p. 5). In addition, there are reports of decreased platelet counts in piglets [80] and altered testicular tissue and steroid hormone levels in miniature pigs [81] fed canola or hydrogenated soybean oil, as well as testicular hyperplasia in boars fed rapeseed oil compared with those fed soybean oil [82].

A clue to the molecular mechanisms of canola oil and hydrogenated oil was obtained in an experiment where mice were fed a diet containing soybean oil, canola oil, or hydrogenated soybean oil together with an essential amount of linoleic acid. A bone morphogenetic protein (BMP) preparation sealed in a sustained-release capsule was then implanted into a gap in the fascia of the right femoral muscle of mice and ectopic bone formation was measured 3 weeks after the implantation. BMPs constitute a group of growth factors originally discovered for their ability to induce bone and cartilage formation. Ectopic formation of new bone was observed at 3 weeks (Figure 10). The volume of newly formed bone was approximately 4-fold greater in the canola and hydrogenated soybean oil groups than in the soybean oil group [83].

Osteocalcin is a non-collagenous protein hormone found in bone. It has glutamyl residues that are γ-carboxylated by an enzyme utilizing vitamin K2 as a co-factor. In its carboxylated form (c-Ocn), it binds calcium directly and thus concentrates in bone, and it is known to suppress BMP-induced formation of ectopic bone. Therefore, the results in Figure 10 are interpreted as follows: VK2-dependent processes were inhibited in the canola and hydrogenated soybean oil groups, both of which exhibited survival-shortening activity in the SHRSP rat (Figure 7, p. 20). In fact, these groups showed a decreased c-Ocn/uc-Ocn ratio compared with the soybean oil group.

Both c-Ocn and uc-Ocn formed in bone are secreted into the bloodstream and serve as bone hormones, targeting organs such as the brain, fat cells, spleen, testis, adrenal gland, and muscle, and later we discuss the impact of inhibition of the VK2-osteocalcin link by some types of vegetable oils on disorders of these organs.

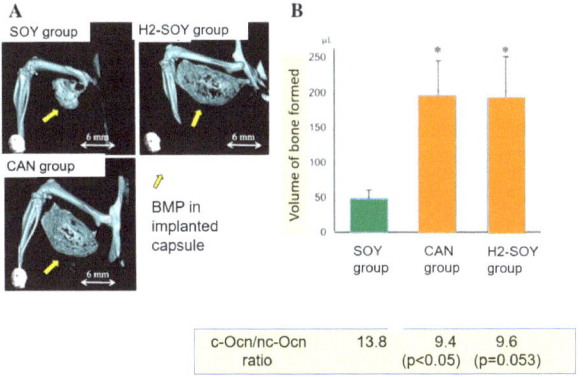

c-Ocn/nc-Ocn ratio	13.8	9.4 (p<0.05)	9.6 (p=0.053)

Figure 10. Newly formed bone in mice fed a soybean oil (Soy), canola oil (Can), or hydrogenated soybean oil (H2-Soy) diet after implantation with a crude extract of BMP. (**a**) Representative reconstructed images generated from 3D R mCT scans of the ectopic newly formed bone (arrow) in the femoral muscle. (**b**) Volume of the newly formed ectopic bone in the three groups of mice calculated from 3D R mCT scans using three-dimensional reconstruction imaging for bone. Figure is reproduced with permission from Ref. [28], with slight modifications. See the text for details. BMPs, bone morphogenetic proteins; 3D R mCT, three-dimensional X-ray micro-computed tomography.

2.3. Hydrogenation of Vegetable Oils Produces Hydrogenated Vitamin K1 (Dihydro-VKI) in Addition to Trans-Fatty Acids, and Clinical Reports Correlate this Process with the VK2–Osteocalcin Link

Partial hydrogenation of polyunsaturated oils is useful in producing fats with desired melting points, but trans-fatty acids are formed as byproducts (hereafter, referred to as industrial trans-fat). Following the proposal by the Harvard U SPH group and other scientists to replace trans-fats with common cis-unsaturated oils, industry in the West responded accordingly. However, the line of evidence behind the proposal was that industrial trans-fat raises the ratio of low- to high-density lipoprotein cholesterol (LDL-C/HDL-C ratio), thereby increasing CHD mortality. However, this line of evidence is not substantiated, as we explained in Chapter 1 and as follows. (1) The association of trans-fat intake with LDL-C level has not been established. Many observational studies failed to demonstrate positive associations. (2) The LDL-C/HDL-C ratio can be readily decreased with medication but no associated decrease in CHD mortality has been reported. High LDL-C is not causative of CHD but is a predictor of longevity among general populations at age ≥50–60 years [10,84]. As shown in Figure 11 (p. 24), a recent meta-analysis to compare industrial trans-fat and ruminant trans-fat (contained in ruminant animals) [85] led to interpretations inconsistent with the mainstream lipid recommendations:

1. All trans-fats and industrial trans-fats but not ruminant trans-fats were associated with increased CHD mortality.
2. Ruminant trans-fats but not all trans-fats were suppressive for diabetes mellitus.

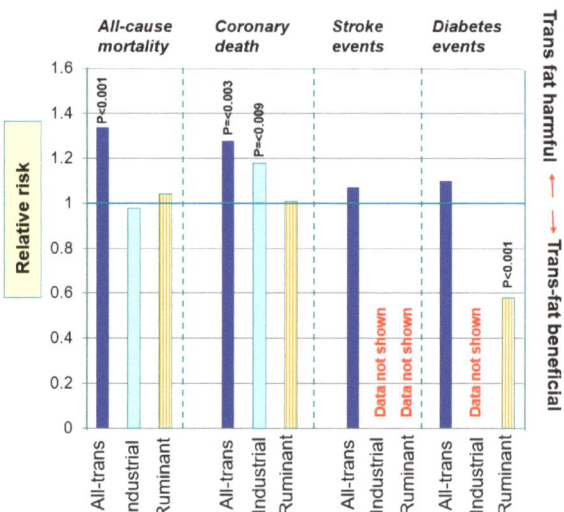

Figure 11. Differential nutritional activity of industrial trans-fats and ruminant trans-fats. Data from Ref. [85] were simplified to emphasize the difference between the two types of trans-fats. See the text for details.

Given that all trans-fats are composed of industrial trans-fats and ruminant trans-fat, reporting only these two results seems to provide an incomplete picture (Figure 11). Additionally, industrial trans-fats may be highly positively associated with diabetes mellitus.

The data shown in Figure 11 cannot be simply explained in terms of the effects on the LDL-C/HDL-C ratio. Rather, we interpret the results as follows [69].

1. Dihydro-VK1 produced during the hydrogenation of vegetable oils is not converted to VK2 and actually interferes with VK2 action, as shown clinically [86,87]. Inhibition of the VK2–osteocalcin link leads to accelerated calcification of the arteries and pancreas, kidney, and other soft organs, resulting in the increased all-cause mortality [69].
2. Foods of ruminant animal origin are enriched with VK2, and VK2 intake as well as plasma VK2 levels are inversely associated with diabetes markers, all-cause mortality, CHD mortality, all cancer mortality, pulmonary cancer, prostate cancer, and bone fracture (Table 2).

Table 2. Clinical studies demonstrating the involvement of VK1, dihydro-VK1, and/or VK2 with the VK2–osteocalcin link.

Population	VK1, Dihydro-Vk1, or WF	VK2	Reference
Healthy	Dihydro-VK1 could not activate Ocn	-	Booth SL, 2001 [86]
Aged population	No correlation	Inverse association of VK2 intake and lumbar bone fracture	Booth SL, 2000 [87]
Healthy postmenopausal women	-	MK-7 supplementation for 3 years, ucOcn/c-Ocn ↓ Loss of vertebrate height ↓	Knapen NH, 2013 [88]
Healthy population	Inverse association of dihydro-VK1 intake with bone mineral density	-	Troy ML [89], 2007
Aged men (RCT)	HOMA-IR lowered with VK1 supplement (500 µg/day, 3 years)	-	Yoshida M, 2008 [90]
Diabetic population	-	VK2 supplementation: Insulin sensitivity ↑, cOcn ↑, ucOcn ↓	Choi HJ, 2011 [91]
Healthy population	No correlation	Inverse association with VK2 intake	Geleijnese JM, 2004 [92]
Hemodialysis patients	No correlation	Warfarin treatment increased bone fracture and aortic calcification	Fusaro M, 2015 [93]
Postmenoposal women with osteoporosis	No correlation	VK2 & VD3 supplementation: bone mineral density ↑	Iwamoto J, 2000 [94]
Heidelberg citizens	No correlation	Inverse associations of VK2 uptake with cancer mortality (pulmonary, prostate, and all sites)	Nmptsch K, 2010 [95]
Chronic kidney disease patients	-	VK2 supplement suppressed decline of bone mineral density	Fusaro M, 2011 [96]
Osteoporosis patients	-	VK supplement:bone fracture ↓, cOcn ↑	Shiraki M, 2000 [97]
Post-menopausal women	-	VK2 (MK-7) supplementation: prevented age-related deterioration of trabecular bone microarchitecture	Rønn SH, 2015 [98]

Abbreviations: cOcn, carboxylated Ocn; HOMA-IR, Homeostatic Model Assessment of Insulin Resistance; ucOcn, under carboxylated Ocn; RCT, randomized controlled trial; VK, vitamin K.

VK1, which is abundant in vegetable oil, is absorbed in various tissues and converted to VK2, which is used as a co-factor of enzyme γ-carboxylating the glutamyl residue of some proteins such as osteocalcin in bone and matrix-Gla protein in soft tissues (Figure 12). Osteocalcin acts as a bone hormone for the target organs shown. Hydrogenation of vegetable oils produces dihydroVK1, which inhibits the VK2–osteocalcin link, leading to the various diseases listed in Table 2. It has also been proposed that the byproduct trans-fat increases the LDL-C/HDL-C ratio, thereby increasing ASCVD [8]. However, we do not believe that this proposal is based on scientific evidence, as explained above.

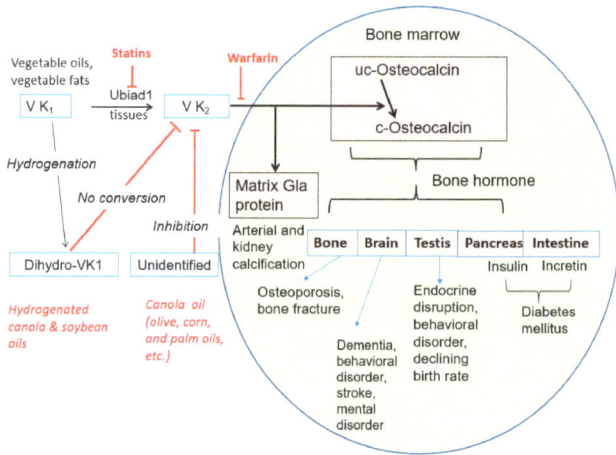

Figure 12. Proposed adverse effects of the two types of byproducts produced during hydrogenation of some types of vegetable oils and vegetable fats known to induce stroke and disrupt endocrines. Figure from Ref. [69] was slightly modified. See the text for details. The substances in red are the inhibitors of the VK2–osteocalcin link. Unidentified, canola oil contains two types of glucosinolates that decompose to form various isothiocyanates (linked to hemorrhagic injury, epithelial cell injury), dimethyl disulfide (hemolytic injury), thiocyanates (linked to rape blindness, psychosis, locomotive disorder) and other substances in animal experiments [99].

2.4. What Differences Could We Expect by Viewing Trans-Fat or Dihydro-VK1 as a Health Risk?

The evidence regarding both trans-fat and dihydro-VK1 leads to the same recommendation—that hydrogenated vegetable oils are not safe. In Western countries, the movement to reduce trans-fat intake was successfully led by industry. However, this movement did not gather much pace in some countries, like Japan. The Japanese government decided not to take any action (in 2018) because the average intake of trans-fat (0.2% of energy) was significantly lower than the WHO recommendation (<1% of energy). In the Japanese market today, margarine and related products still occupy greater space than butter does, despite our recommendation. When the fats and oils industry in Western countries recognized that palm oil was less expensive and was almost trans-fat-free compared with hydrogenated vegetable oils, the consumption of palm oil increased rapidly in these countries. Alongside these positive changes, however, the problems of dihydro-VKI and unidentified components in canola, olive, and some other vegetable oils have been disregarded.

In producing edible palatable palm oil, higher refining temperatures are used, and 3-MCPD (3-monochloro-propane diol) is formed from oil derivatives and chlorine. The WHO/FAO Joint Expert Committee on Food Additives[4] and specialists in many countries studied this minor component for decades [100]. We estimated that the daily intake/TDI ratios for 3-MCPD are currently 1 for the general population and 2.5 for infants in Japan. The ratio is higher in infants because palm oil contains greater amounts of 3-MCPD than most other fats and oils and is selectively used in infant formula. In calculating TDI, we applied the uncertainty coefficients (safety coefficients) of 0.1 (difference between species), 0.1 (difference between individuals in a species), and 0.5 (to account for reproduction and generation-related toxicity). Based on this result, the WHO/FAO Joint Expert Committee on Food Additives advised reducing 3-MCPD in cooking oils.

While it may be relatively easy to solve this 3-MCPD problem, as lowering temperature and NaCl availability during the refining process helps in reducing them, there are more serious health problems associated with ingesting vegetable fats and oils that still need to be tackled. The toxicity of canola oil and hydrogenated oils is a much more serious issue, as we can see when we estimate this using the same uncertainty coefficients we used for 3-MCPD.

Compared with soybean oil, canola oil and hydrogenated soybean oil both exhibited stroke-inducing, survival-shortening, and testosterone-reducing activity in SHRSP rats (Chapter 2). DNA microarray analysis of rat testis revealed that >80% of the genes affected were common to the canola oil and hydrogenated oil groups, and the degree of the altered ratio (vs. soybean oil group) was quantitively similar. While the principles of toxicity are different between unidentified components in the canola oil and dihydro-VK1 in the hydrogenated soybean oil, their toxicity to the testis is likely to be similar. Although dose-response in this study was investigated only for a soybean oil/canola oil mixture, canola oil accounting for as little as 6% of energy significantly reduced survival. Hence, the TDI value is calculated to be <0.033% of energy if we apply the same method of calculation used for 3-MCPD (uncertainty factors of $0.1 \times 0.1 \times 0.5$). Canola oil intake is actually estimated to account for 5.7%

---

[4] See http://www.fao.org/food/food-safety-quality/scientific-advice/jecfa/en/ (accessed on 28 September 2020).

of energy in the Japanese population. The impact of canola oil on the population is therefore roughly estimated to be 170-fold greater than that of 3-MCPD. Besides canola oil, other oils such as olive oil, corn oil, palm oil, and oleic-rich safflower and sunflower oils have all exhibited survival-shortening activity [21,41,76,77]. Therefore, the impact of these oils on human nutrition should no longer be disregarded as it has been for decades. Moreover, it should be noted that animal fats are much safer in these stroke-prone rats, which is in line with the evidence obtained from clinical studies that cholesterol and saturated animal fats are beneficial for the prevention of stroke [16,101–104]. Industrial trans-fat is likely to be a surrogate marker of dihydro-VK1, so it is imperative that the Japanese administrative authorities and the food industry urgently re-evaluate the safety of industrial trans-fat given its known stroke-inducing and endocrine-disrupting activity (Figure 12, p. 26).

In this section, we also want to emphasize that the increase in vegetable oil intake in Japan was followed by increased incidence of ASCVD and other lifestyle-related diseases (/10^5 population, not age-adjusted). Separately from plasma LDL-C and other cholesterol-related parameters, some types of vegetable fats and oils have been shown to induce atherogenesis by inhibiting the VK2–osteocalcin link and to induce arterial calcification [16,28,69].

Statins and warfarin both inhibit VK2 formation, so long-term administration likely induces atherosclerosis. Statins also directly inhibit the conversion of VK1 to VK2 [105]. On the other hand, many types of antimicrobial drugs were developed based on the selectivity that nuclear DNA and protein synthesis in animal cells is more resistant than bacterial DNA and protein synthesis. However, mitochondrial DNA and protein synthesis in animal cells is similarly sensitive to these drugs and mitochondrial protein synthesis is likely inhibited, possibly resulting in impaired matrix protein synthesis and greater frailty of blood vessels. In fact, the fluoroquinoline group of antimicrobial drugs increases aortic dissection 2.79-fold and aortic aneurysms 2.25-fold [106]. Extracellular collagen synthesis is also impaired, leading to increased Achilles tendon breakage. The macrolide group of antibacterial drugs exhibit similar adverse effects on brain function, in addition to aortic intima-media dissociation, Achilles tendon cleavage, and increased CHD mortality [107]. The adverse effects after two months of antimicrobial drug use appear to last for more than a year.

In this section, we have summarized three mechanisms of atherogenesis independent of plasma cholesterol: (1) some types of vegetable fats and oils inhibit the VK2–osteocalcin link, resulting in accelerated artery calcification; (2) statins and warfarin inhibit VK2 synthesis and reactivation of VK2, resulting in inhibition of the VK2–osteocalcin link; and (3) inhibition of mitochondrial DNA and protein synthesis by some types of antibacterial drugs increases the frailty of blood vessels by decreasing intercellular matrix protein synthesis.

Chapter 2 Summary

Some kinds of vegetable fats and oils were demonstrated to be toxic to SHRSP rats, inducing pathological changes in the brain and kidney, decreasing platelet counts, inducing stroke, and shortening survival time by 40%. The active components in canola oil have not been identified, but they are transferred to offspring. In the case of hydrogenated oils, dihydro-VK1 is interpreted to be a causative factor. These oils were found to inhibit the VK2–osteocalcin (Ocn) link, sharing the same mechanisms of action as statins and warfarin [69]. Because Ocn acts as a bone hormone targeting organs such as the brain, intestine, and testis, these oils and drugs exert toxic effects on many organs. This is supported by increasing numbers of clinical reports reporting the correlation of this mechanism with lifestyle-related disease. These lines of evidence indicate that atherogenesis can develop without elevated LDL-C levels and/or in association with decreasing LDL-C levels.

3. Industry-Oriented Lipid Nutritional Guidelines Have Likely Endangered Some Populations

3.1. Changes in Lipid Nutrition Are Consistent with Changes in Disease Patterns in Japan

Around 1965–1975 in Japan, the intake of vegetable oils and animal fats increased 3-fold as the livestock industry successfully utilized oilseeds such as corn, soybean, and canola/rapeseed on a large scale. These industrial changes occurred roughly 5 years after they were introduced in some Western countries, and many other countries later followed suit. The incidence of diabetes and chronic kidney disease started to increase around 1980 along with decreases in total energy and carbohydrate energy intake. In animal experiments, intake of some types of vegetable oils was shown to be associated with the development of diabetes and kidney disease as well as mental disorders (Table 1). Statin use became popular after 1990, so its contribution to the increased incidence of diabetes and kidney disease shown in Figure 13 may not be a major factor. The number of patients with mental illness began to increase from around 1995, suggesting that the exposure to toxic fats and oils early in life (e.g., during in utero and neonatal development) is more critical in the development of mental diseases than in the development of diabetes and kidney disease.

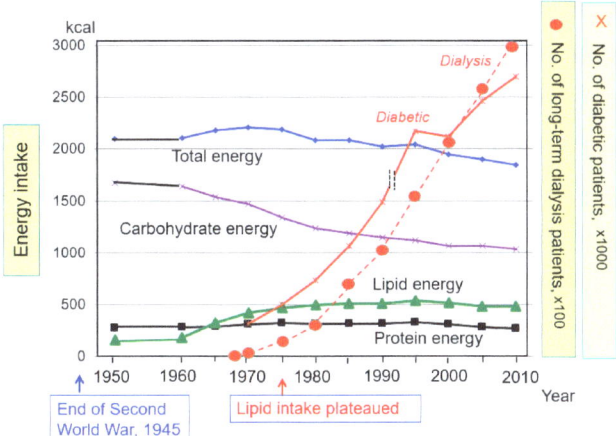

Figure 13. Trends in Japanese nutrient intake and the numbers of patients on long-term dialysis or with diabetes mellitus. Figure 11 in Ref. [69] was modified to include a dataset for chronic dialysis patients. See the text for more details.

Here, we would like to emphasize the consistent correlation of changes in lipid nutrition and changes in many types of diseases in Japan, suggesting a causal relationship. In the USA, decreased total lipid intake is associated with increased incidence of diabetes and increased intake of carbohydrates, but the intake of vegetable oils is unlikely to have decreased over the past several decades because of the powerful campaign to increase vegetable oil intake by government authorities, medical societies, and leading nutritionists.

3.2. The People of Hisayama Town Were Misled by Nutritionists Unquestioningly Following the Mainstream Recommendations

Dietary recommendations in Japan were guided by a team at Kyushu University School of Agriculture who essentially adopted the recommendations made by WHO and the Harvard U SPH group. Moreover, the administrative agencies of Japan emphasized that the risk of hydrogenated vegetable oil was negligible in the amounts ingested, so strong recommendations were made from the 1960s onward to increase the polyunsaturated/saturated ratio of ingested lipids together with soy isoflavones. At this time, Kyushu University School of Medicine teamed up with the town leaders and residents of Hisayama Town to conduct long-term research [108]. The chiefs of the medical and nutrition teams from the Kyushu University School of Medicine and from the National Cerebral and Cardiovascular Center in Osaka, Japan, appear to have been convinced that the residents had very good health status, but over time the residents themselves came to reach a different conclusion. At the 30th anniversary of the commencement of the Hisayama Study, the former Mayor, Arata Kobayakawa, who collaborated with the medical teams and nutritionists to start the study, conveyed the following to the townspeople [109] (Kobayakawa A, 1993, translated into English by us): "Despite the considerable efforts that we have made so far, the number of sick people has increased. So, you should look after your health yourself."

Mr. Kobayakawa did not leave actual data for us to review, but we characterized the health status of Hisayama residents as follows: (1) a 2-fold higher prevalence of diabetes mellitus compared with people in Funagata Town who received no special dietary advice [110]; (2) extremely high stroke mortality and the highest among nine selected cities across the world [28]; and (3) prevalent cognitive disorders among those aged ≥65 years, which in 2017 was top among the member countries of the Organization for Economic Co-operation and Development [111][5]. The leader of the Hisayama study at the Kyushu Uuniversity School of Medicine reported on his homepage an extremely high incidence of subarachnoid hemorrhage in Hisayama

---

[5] See https://doi.org/10.1787/health_glance-2017-en (accessed on 28 September 2020).

residents compared with several other countries (Framingham, USA; Tartu, Estonia; Izumo, Japan; Helsinki, Finland; Carlisle, UK; Ireland; Shibata, Japan) [28], although unfortunately we are not able to reproduce one of the figures here.

The mechanism that we propose to explain the tragedy for Hisayama residents is that some types of vegetable fats and oils accelerated these diseases by inhibiting the VK2–osteocalcin link.

Figure 14 shows our calculations using food intake data for Hisayama residents and the general Japanese population for the 60–70 years age group. The food intake of Hisayama residents [112,113] was not different from that of the average Japanese population in terms of total energy intake or energy percent of total protein, total lipids, or carbohydrates. However, Hisayama residents had a higher intake of vegetable fats and oils (69.4% vs. 51%) and a lower intake of animal protein (37.4% vs. 51%). The vegetable oil/animal fat ratio was roughly 1:2 for Hisayama residents compared with 1/1 for the average Japanese population. These differences in the quality of ingested lipids and proteins are consistent with our proposed mechanisms for the onset of diabetes, stroke, and dementia (Figure 12, p. 26). Thus, the current mainstream recommendations on lipid nutrition being given to Hisayama residents need to be reversed—they should be told that animal fats are, in fact, relatively safe and are beneficial for the prevention of stroke and other lifestyle-related diseases.

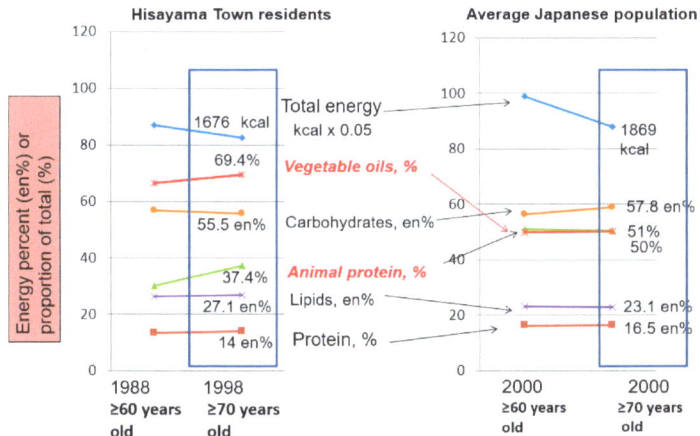

Figure 14. Comparison of nutrient intake between Hisayama Town residents and the average Japanese population. Figure shows data for calculations made based on data from Ref. [113] and the National Nutrition Survey [114].

Another issue we want to discuss here is how medical staff from Kyushu University School of Medicine and the National Cerebral and Cardiovascular Center tried to convince Hisayama residents that the medications provided had been successful in promoting health. However, former Mayor Kobayakawa left important messages that some patients were moved to other (university) hospitals outside the study area, which showed residents to have better data than they actually did. Also, the life expectancy of the residents was recalculated to exclude some of the disabled residents to show better life expectancy than for the average Japanese population. This immoral manipulation of the data prompted the former mayor to ultimately advise residents to be responsible for their own health. After that, some residents started turning to herbal medicine [28].

It should be noted that the National Cerebral and Cardiovascular Center is a branch of the Ministry of Health, Labour and Welfare, Japan. Findings from follow-up studies on plasma cholesterol and cerebro- and cardiovascular diseases (Nippon DATA collected by this Center) were used as the major basis for the Cholesterol Guidelines issued by the Japan Atherosclerosis Society, on which our cholesterol-lowering medications in Japan depend. We have found many scientific problems associated with Nippon DATA and the Cholesterol Guidelines; as described in detail elsewhere [10,19]. Most of the Japanese population are still not aware that, in fact, high plasma cholesterol is a predictor of longevity, that statins' cholesterol-lowering activity is not associated with decreased CHD mortality, and that statins can increase cerebro- and cardiovascular disease as well as several other lifestyle-related diseases by inhibiting the VK2–osteocalcin link.

3.3. International Differences in Population and Health Status Are Potentially Associated with Lipid Nutrition

In this chapter so far, we have focused mainly on the relationship between lipid nutrition and health in the Japanese population. Here, we start to broaden our discussion to include the relationship observed in other populations across the world, as well as look at how some populations trends could be associated with lipid nutrition.

Japanese people have long enjoyed the status of having among the highest average life expectancy in the world, and the administrative authorities have confirmed that their healthy life expectancy is also among the highest. However, according to the World Population Prospects from the United Nations [28,115], while the population is steadily increasing in many Western countries, this is not at all the case in Japan, where its declining birth rate tops the world. In the worst case, Japan's population will decrease to half its present level by 2100 (Figure 15) [28,115]. In the best case, when the cause of this population change is defined, it will take half a century for this trend to stop and for the population rate to stabilize.

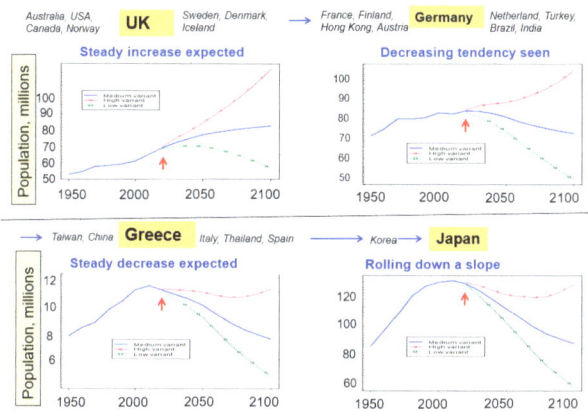

Figure 15. Comparison of trends in population changes among countries and regions of the world. Figure is from Ref. [28].

The original set of data was based on those reported from United Nations DESA/Population Division, World Population Prospects 2017 [115], the countries and area were selected by us and recorded as shown here [28]. Similar tendency has been reported for Japanese by Morisaki Nao et al. [116], predicting that the Japanese population would be half its current size in 2100, and at 10% of the current level after 200 years. Since around 1980, the birth rate has decreased, the low birth weight rate has increased, and average height among young Japanese has decreased [116], as discussed later in this chapter.

This century, the populations of the UK, USA, and northern EU countries are expected to increase steadily, while those of Germany and the Netherlands among other countries show a tendency toward decline. Mediterranean countries such as Greece and Italy show rates of population decline almost as obvious as that of Japan's. Similar trends in population decline are seen among a number of East Asian countries, including Japan, mainland China, Taiwan (China), and Korea.

We know that it is imprudent to try to correlate lipid nutrition with the different trends in population change seen in different countries, because many other factors are at play, such as socio-economic, religious, medicinal, and political factors. However, we do want to bring natural science into the discussion about the declining birth rates in many countries and regions.

As we mentioned in Section 2.1, Ratnayake's group [76,77] reported that olive oil exhibited survival-shortening activity in SHRSP rats. Olive oil and canola oil are common in the Mediterranean, as canola oil is in East Asia, and these trends may contribute to the low birth rates observed in these areas. Another factor possibly associated with the low birth rate is the rate of low birth weight babies. In Japan, the low birth weight rate decreased after the Second World War but began to rise after around 1980 (Figure 16).

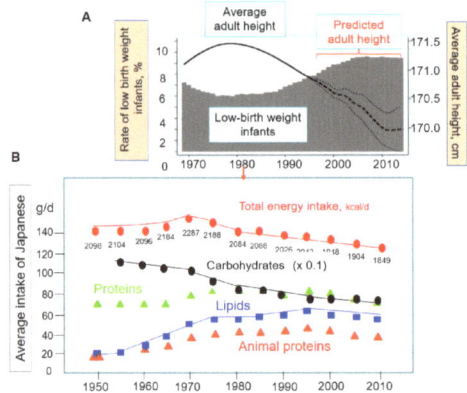

Figure 16. A pivotal point seen at around 1980 in the trends of low birth weight infants and nutrient intake. (**A**) Trends in the rates of low birth weight babies (<2500 g) and adult height in Japan. Figure based on data kindly provided by Dr. Morisaki, 2017 [116]. See the text for details. The rate of low birth weight infants (1969–2014, gray bars), average adult height (1969–1996, solid line), and predicted adult height (1997–2014, dotted line) are shown by year of birth among men. Data for women were similar (not shown). (**B**) Change in average intake of different nutrients over a longer period in the Japanese population [28].

Obviously, the trend here is not parallel with the number of cases of maternal undernutrition. On the other hand, Japanese people who saw American troops after the Second World War were astonished by how tall they were. Today, young Japanese people have reached the height of Americans at that time; that is, Japanese height increased from the post-war period up until 1980 (Figure 16), before decreasing again, and this decreasing trend is predicted to continue. The estimated decrease in Japanese height is only 1.5 cm, but the value is accurate because it is based on 64 million people. Again, changes in lipid nutrition (a 3-fold increase during 1965–1975) are likely to have contributed to this decrease in height, given that the sequence of events is consistent with the causality seen in animal experiments where the growth of offspring was affected by the lipid intake of the dams (Figure 9, p. 21). Interestingly, Japan and Greece have the highest low birth weight rates (Figure 15). In this context, we pay attention to the results of the Helsinki Birth Cohort Study, where it was found that pre-term birth is associated with an increased risk of type 2 diabetes in adult life (the risk is independent of that associated with slow fetal growth (odds ratio: 1.59 [117]) and also that the risk of severe mental disorders across adulthood has increased among individuals born small and among individuals born post-term [118].

Increased mental health disorders in Japan after around 1990 will be commented on later.

Another aspect of lipid nutrition related to ASCVD is that dietary cholesterol and animal fats were found to be protective for stroke and not to promote CHD in observational clinical studies (as described above). After the Second World War, Japanese people living in cold northeastern areas had a significantly lower average lifespan due to high mortality from stroke. People believed the explanation that high salt intake from salted pickles was the cause of hypertension and apoplexy. However, a group of epidemiologists led by the late Professor Yoshio Komachi (University of Tsukuba) revealed that it was not high intake of salt but low intake of animal fats and proteins that explained the hypertension and apoplexy [119].

Animal experiments, mainly performed in SHRSP rats, provided consistent results, and the mechanism has been clarified in part. Some vegetable oils that are commonly used worldwide can induce the onset of stroke, but dietary cholesterol and saturated fats do not and they appear to strengthen cerebral artery vessels, even though the brain can synthesize saturated fats and cholesterol (Figures 7–10 in Chapter 2 and Figure 17) [10,16–19,68,69,75–79,120,121].

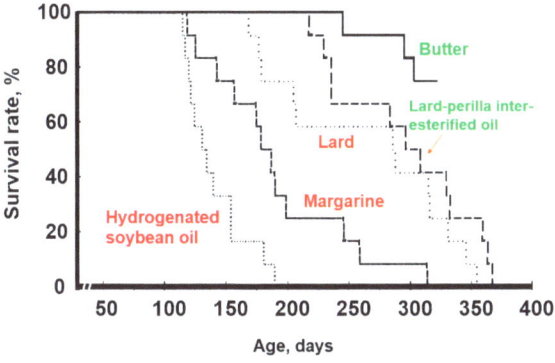

Figure 17. Evaluation of animal fats and trans-fat in SHRSP rats. Experimental conditions were the same as in Figure 7 [75]. Lard and soybean oil diets showed similar survival times. Margarine bought from a local market contained hydrogenated vegetable oil. A mixture of lard and perilla oil was treated with lipase to obtain an inter-esterified oil. Figure is based on data from Ref. [121].

Our recommendation to increase and not to reduce the intake of animal fats for the prevention of ischemic and hemorrhagic stroke is based both on the clinical observational studies listed above and on animal experiments (Figure 17). Animal fats do not have detectable stroke-inducing or endocrine-disrupting activity, but some types of vegetable fats and oils do and they inhibit the VK2–osteocalcin link, leading to stroke and other diseases.

Based on these new observations, we compared current trends and changes in stroke in different areas of the world [122,123], as cited in Figures 18 and 19. The risk of stroke was found to differ greatly among countries and regions (Figures 18 and 19). The stroke risk in the period 1990–2016 (green bars in Figure 19) shows a decreasing tendency in eastern Europe only, which may be due to increasing intake of animal foods including animal fats in this region. Conversely, the increasing trend of stroke is remarkable in East Asia.

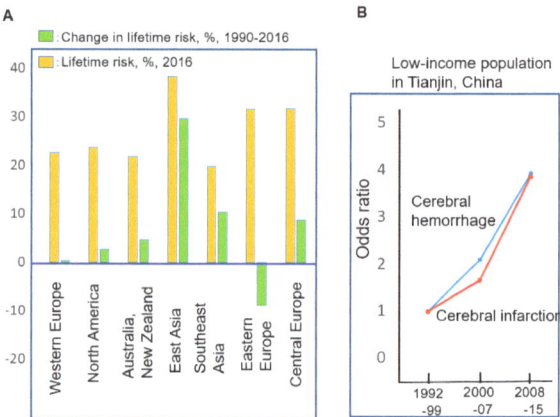

Figure 18. The lifetime risk of stroke and changes across the world and in a low-income population in China. (**A**) Men and women age >25 years were followed during 1990–2016 in the Global Burden of Disease Study. Figure is based on data from Ref. [122]. (**B**) A low-income population in Tianjin, China, was followed from 1992 for 24 years [123] and stroke (ischemic and hemorrhagic) morbidity (age-adjusted) increased from 122 to 216/100,000 people. Figure is based on data from Ref. [123].

In a rural low-income population in Tianjin, China (Figure 18b), 14,920 residents (aged 35–64 years) were registered and followed for 24 years (1992–2015). The odds ratio of stroke increased from 1 (1992–1999) to 4 (2008–2015) for both ischemic and hemorrhagic types (Figure 19b). The burden of stroke in China was described to originate primarily in young and middle-aged adults [123].

In terms of the type of lipids ingested by Chinese adults, the ratio of vegetable oils to animal fats was extremely high in 1980 and has only been increasing (Figure 19), reaching 20/1 among residents of urban areas and 5/1 among residents of rural farming villages in 2012. In the case of Japanese adults, the ratio has remained roughly 1/1 for the past several decades. The high ratio of dietary vegetable oils to animal fats is thus a risk factor for stroke, as we have repeatedly explained and as evidenced by the Hisayama Study in Japan (Figure 14, p. 33) [28].

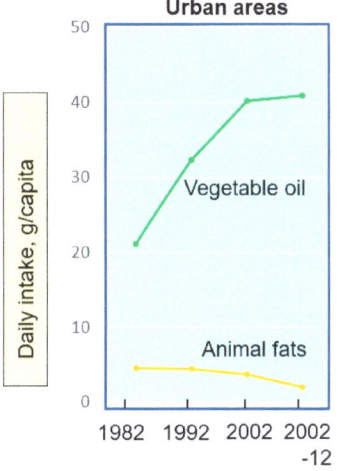 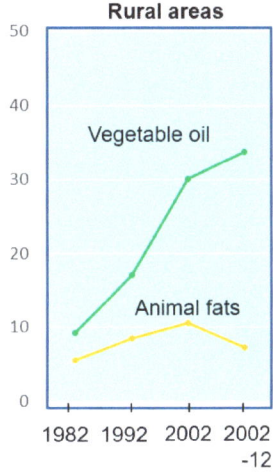

Figure 19. Trend in fat and oil intake in Chinese men (age ≥18 years). Average intake of energy is 2400 kcal/capita. The vegetable oil/animal fat ratio is much higher than in the average populations of Japan and European countries (Figures 14 and 18). Figure is based on data from Ref. [124].

Stroke incidence is likely to be affected by the balance of intake of animal fats vs. vegetable fats and oils, particularly those that exhibit toxic effects on SHRSP rats. Unfortunately, an accurate intake dataset has not been available to us, but the major vegetable oils consumed in some countries are shown in Figure 20 (p. 40). It should be noted that the consumption includes the amounts used for foods and non-foods, and the amounts of hydrogenated fats are not known. Non-food use of butter and cheese is relatively small, so they can serve as good markers of the intake of animal fats and VK2, respectively. It is interesting to note that the three countries defeated in the Second World War (Japan, Italy, and Germany) share the feature of population decline and a high prevalence of cognitive disorder, although we cannot reach any definitive conclusions from these data as to why. We return to this point later in Chapter 4.

In Japan, a further concern is that among the two or three soybean varieties available, almost all of the soybean oil supplied for use in schools is prepared from genetically modified varieties. This is despite no safety evaluations having been conducted using SHRSP rats, because the oils from different varieties are not available to do so. The lack of more accurate data on the consumption of different types of fats and oils in different countries and regions is an urgent matter to address.

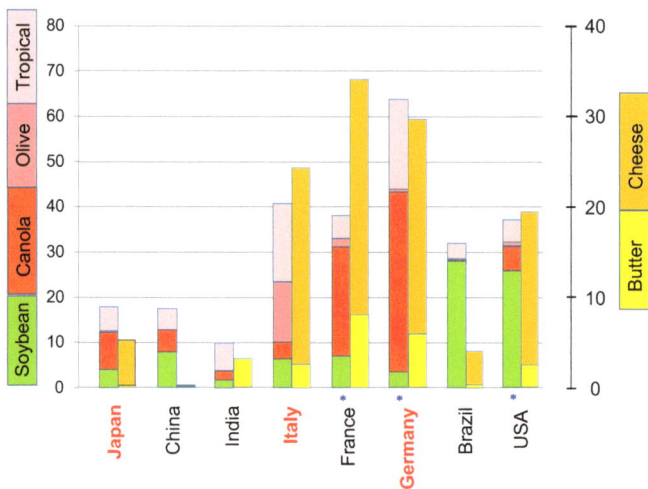

Figure 20. Annual consumption of fats and oils (kg/capita) in different countries. Among EU countries, 63% of the annual canola oil production (9.39 million tons) is used for biofuel. Asterisks indicate countries conducting advanced research on the industrial use of canola oil. The original source of the diary consumption data (butter and cheese) is the Japan Dairy Association (j-milk) [125]. The oil data (soybean, canola, olive and tropical) was gathered from an online search of 556 specialized dictionaries, Japanese dictionaries and encyclopedias [126]. Note: This figure and accompanying sources were updated on 15 July 2024 to better reflect the data collected by the authors.

3.4. Some Types of Vegetable Oils with Endocrine-Disrupting Activity Affect Sexual Development and Physical and Mental Disorders

Let's look specifically now at how the consumption of certain vegetable oils that have endocrine-disrupting activity may influence not only sexual development, but also the development of physical and mental disorders, and the impact of such consumption in different countries around the world.

Among the types of vegetable oils that have shown stroke-inducing activity, canola oil and hydrogenated oil have been examined repeatedly for their endocrine-disrupting activity. In male SHRSP rats, we found significantly lower testis and plasma levels of testosterone in the canola oil and hydrogenated soybean oil groups compared with the soybean oil group [127] (Figure 21).

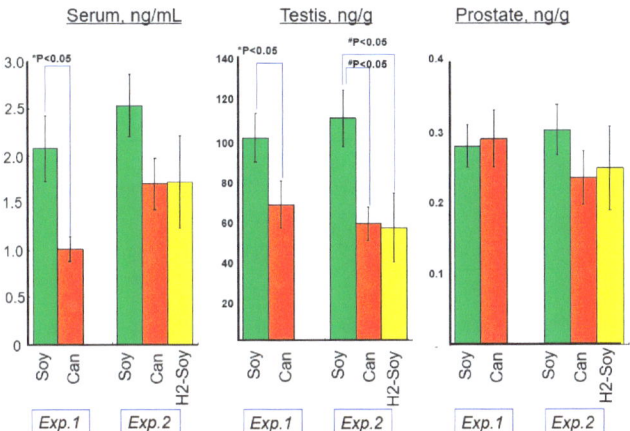

Figure 21. Suppression of tissue testosterone levels by dietary canola oil (Can) and hydrogenated soybean oil (H2-Soy) compared with soybean oil (Soy). Male SHRSP rats raised without NaCl-loading were sacrificed at 16 weeks of age and the tissue samples excised were kept frozen until analysis. Deuterated testosterone was used as an internal standard, and testosterone was quantified with an LC/MS/MS apparatus [127]. Figure reproduced with permission from Ref. [127], with slight modifications to add data for male animals in Experiment 1.

Dihydro-VK1 in the hydrogenated soybean oil and unidentified alkaline-sensitive components in the canola oil inhibited the VK2–osteocalcin link, as explained in Figure 12 (p. 26). Both carboxylated osteocalcin (c-Ocn) and non-carboxylated osteocalcin (nc-Ocn) are released from bone into the bloodstream. According to Oury et al. [128,129], both forms bind to Leydig cells to stimulate testosterone synthesis, and this is accompanied by up-regulation of StAR, Cyp11, Cyp17, and 3-HSD [130]. Testosterone stimulates sperm production and suppresses apoptosis of sperm in the spermatocytes. Thus, with increased intake of canola oil and hydrogenated vegetable oils after 1965–1975, the Japanese population has been exposed to endocrine disruptors from vegetable fats and oils over the long term. Statins and warfarin share the same mechanism of VK2–osteocalcin link inhibition [68].

More than a couple of decades ago, we heard that young men's semen had become thinner. Soon after, specialists in this field confirmed such changes in many countries, with one specialist warning in 2008 that the adverse trends seen in male reproductive health indicated that "we may have reached a crucial tipping point" [131]. A survey of young Japanese men revealed that they may have significantly worse sperm properties than young men in some European countries [132] (Figure 22, p. 42). This could be related to the fact that Japanese people are exposed to the largest amounts of vegetable fats and oils with endocrine-disrupting activity (170-fold greater potential compared with the widely recognized most potent dioxin, polychlorinated dibenzofuran, the tetra chlorinated form).

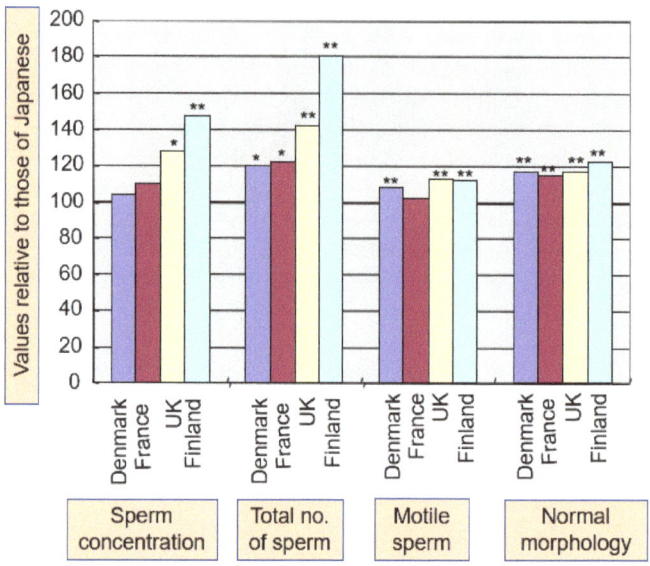

Figure 22. Sperm properties of fertile Japanese men (n = 324) compared with some European counterparts. Data kindly provided by one of the authors, Dr. Teruaki Iwamoto, of Ref. [132]. * $p < 0.02$, ** $p < 0.0002$.

Also, what would be the effects of the inhibition of testosterone synthesis on pregnancy? Testosterone is synthesized from cholesterol abundantly in the testis, but it is also synthesized in several other organs, including the brain. Interestingly, it is converted to estrogens, typical female steroid hormones, and exerts effects through estrogen receptors, in a process common to both sexes. Genetic sex is determined at mating: it is female when the fertilized egg contains XX chromosomes and is male when it contains XY chromosomes. In the case of XY, when the fertilized egg starts dividing and proliferating, the sex-determining region on the Y chromosome is activated to form testosterone, which activates the development of male internal and external genitalia (Figure 23). In the case of XX, estrogens from the gonadal apparatus activate the development of female internal and external genitalia and testosterone is not essential in this process. Hence, the inhibitors of testosterone synthesis, including several types of vegetable fats and oils, are likely to affect the development of male sexual characteristics much more than female sexual characteristics within the first 10 weeks of gestation.

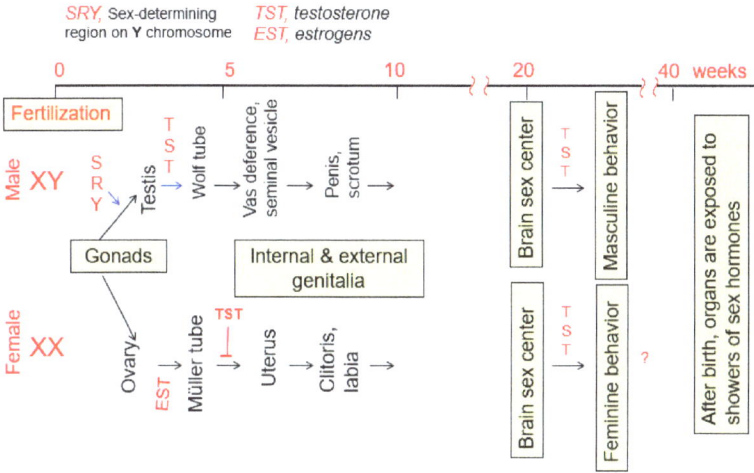

Figure 23. Explanatory scheme of sex differentiation during the human lifecycle and potential to affect development of male and female behavior. See the text for details.

After 20 weeks of gestation, the amount of testosterone synthesized in the sex center of the brain appears to affect the development of male and female behavior. Even after birth, testosterone and estrogens must be produced in adequate amounts at appropriate times in the brain and other sexual organs in order for bearers of XY and XX chromosomes to develop masculine and feminine properties. Any disorder in these processes may potentially have some involvement in the development of gender dysphoria.

It is worth noting that there is a greater proportion of women than men in the Japanese population that has been long exposed to some vegetable oils exhibiting endocrine-disrupting activity. The female/male ratio at birth is known to be about 0.95, but in the general Japanese population, it has been 1.06 for many years. Although the countries that were defeated in the Second World War exhibit a similar tendency (female/male ratio of 1.04–1.07 for Germany, Japan, and Italy), this gender imbalance is not seen in Sweden and Norway (1.00–1.01) where populations are predicted to increase steadily toward the next generation (Figure 15, p. 35) [28]. Needless to say, it may well be premature to correlate gender imbalance and disorders of sexual development to lipid nutrition based on the evidence we have so far, but the possibility should be kept in mind as evidence continues to accumulate.

In terms of generational effects of vegetable oils, as mentioned earlier, when we raised SHRSP rats on a soybean oil or canola oil diet, mated them at 12 weeks of age (F0), and weaned the offspring (F1) to the same diet as dams at 4 weeks of age or to a different diet, the survival of the F1 generation was shortened not only by their own diet, but also by the diet consumed by their parents (Figure 9, p. 21) [80]. It appears that the survival-shortening factor present in the canola oil (the breakdown products of two kinds of glucosinolates) is transferred to the offspring via the umbilical vein, as lipophilic materials are generally known to be transferred, and there is no reason to believe that human beings are exceptional in this regard.

We have also reported that two generational feedings of high-linoleic safflower oil or perilla oil with a high α-linolenic/linoleic acid ratio affected learning and memory as well as general behavioral patterns in various strains of rats (Table 1, p. 5). In addition, when we fed groups of mice a diet containing different vegetable oils for a relatively long period (corn, canola, soybean, safflower, perilla, and a mixture of perilla and safflower oils), the canola oil group exhibited significantly different behavioral patterns, which could not be accounted for by the difference in the n-6/n-3 balance [133]. They exhibited much higher locomotor activity, higher ambulation activity, higher rearing activity, faster acquisition in the water maze task, and slower habituation behavior compared with the soybean oil group.

Such studies are not easy to perform clinically, but many types of behavioral problems associated with cognitive and mental disorders are frequently reported in Japan and the incidence is increasing (Figure 24). Whereas the incidence of epilepsy, mental retardation, and autonomic neuropathy has remained relatively unchanged or has been decreasing, for which genetic factors are assumed to be deeply involved, the incidence of depression, insomnia, Alzheimer's disease, Parkinsonism, and autism has been increasing rapidly, for which environmental factors seem to play important roles, given that genetic factors do not change much over decades.

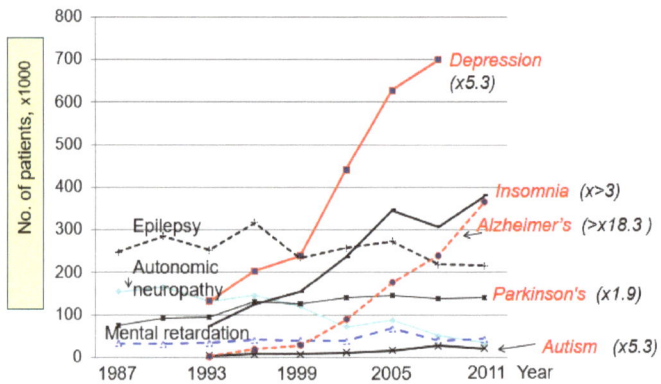

Figure 24. Trends in the incidence of mental disorders in Japan. Figure is based on data from the 2017 List of Statistical Surveys conducted by Ministry of Health, Labour and Welfare, Japan [134]. Numbers in parentheses denote x-fold increases during this period.

While we recognize that one of the major reasons for the increased number of patients with mental disorders recorded in Japan is probably the ease with which physicians have been able to prescribe new medications developed over the last two decades, such as donepezil for Alzheimer's disease, SSRIs for depression, and zolpidem for insomnia, we also want to emphasize that the intake of vegetable oils (1965–1975) preceded this increased use of psychotropic drugs. Moreover, this sequence of events is the same for diabetes, kidney disease, and other dietary lipid-related diseases.

It could be argued that cognitive disorders are inevitable as they are associated with aging. When Japan was first reported to top the OECD countries in prevalence of cognitive disorders, we simply interpreted this as reasonable, given the long average life expectancy of Japanese people and the assumption that cognitive disorders are naturally more prevalent in aged societies (Figure 25). However, the facts may be different.

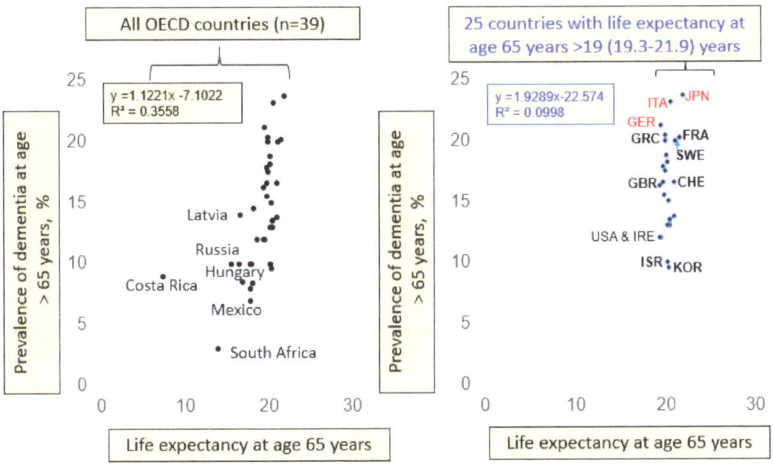

Figure 25. Prevalence of cognitive disorders among the OECD countries for 2017. Figure is based on data from Ref. [134]. Japan ranks number one among these countries and this cannot be explained by differences in "aging rate" alone. See the text for details. The prevalence of cognitive disorders for Japan is reported to be based on the Hisayama Study [65], a value which was 1.5-fold higher than that given in governmental statistics reports (15.2–15.6%) for 2015 [134]. The three countries shown in red, including Japan, are those which were defeated in the Second World War.

First, we want to point out that average life expectancy at age 65 years is not much different between the OECD countries, at 20±1.5 years for most countries. Even though Japan often ranks top for average life expectancy, the standard population pyramids used in different countries are likely to differ (Figure 25) and the difference in average life expectancy at 0 years of age among countries may be smaller. Also, the standard population pyramids shown for different countries in Figure 26 are based on 1985 data, and the current population pyramid for Japan has a much smaller proportion of younger generations. Specialists in this field may criticize this kind of speculation, but the shapes of standard population pyramids are diverse and they change at different speeds in different countries, and age-adjusted data may not be as accurate as we used to believe. Second, when we look at the OECD's data on the prevalence of dementia, it is reported only for the proportion of the population aged ≥65 years (Figure 25).

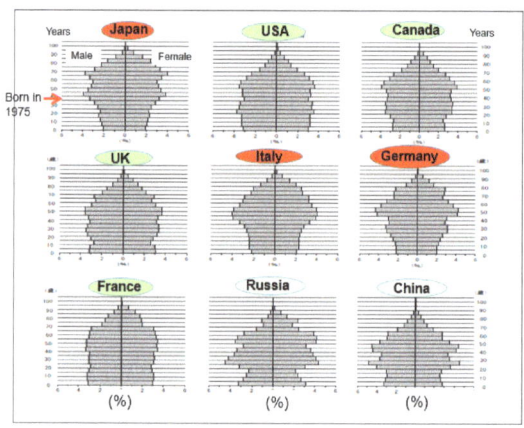

Figure 26. Differences in standard population pyramids among selected countries. Figure is from Ref. [28]. Data are from 2015 except for Japan, where data are from 2017. The three countries shown in red are those defeated in the Second World War.

When we take the 25 countries with life expectancy at 65 years of >19 years, we find essentially no positive correlation of dementia prevalence with life expectancy at 65 years of age (Figure 25, $R^2 = 0.0998$). Thus, the difference in average life expectancy at age 65 (85 ± 1.5 years) among different countries would seem unlikely to explain the large difference seen in prevalence of dementia between Japan at 24% and Korea at <10%.

3.5. The Wrong Lipid Nutrition Is Potentially Endangering the Japanese People

Since around 1965, 20 years after the Second World War ended, Japanese people have followed authoritative lipid nutrition guidelines, increasing their intake of vegetable oils in place of animal fats. When many countries started regulating hydrogenated vegetable oils for safety reasons, the Japanese government took no regulatory action. The major types of vegetable oils consumed in Japan today are canola rapeseed oil, palm oil, olive oil, and hydrogenated-soybean and -canola oil [28], and Japanese people have a much lower intake of animal fats than their Western counterparts. This is despite the mechanisms of these vegetable oils to exert toxicity having already been partly clarified (see Chapter 2 and Section 3.4). Specifically, the dihydro-VK1 produced during the hydrogenation of vegetable oils inhibits the conversion of VK1 to VK2 and also inhibits the VK2-dependent activities of osteocalcin (in bone), matrix-Gla protein (in soft tissues), and other similar proteins. The target organs of these hormones are diverse, including the brain, testis, pancreas, and intestine, and hence the consequences of vegetable oils inhibiting these processes are diverse (Figure 13, p. 31). As cholesterol-lowering medicines, statins inhibit VK2 formation via a mechanism common to that of these vegetable oils. Moreover, statins inhibit the formation of (iso)prenyl intermediates and protein glycosylation, therefore inhibiting other steps in cellular metabolism [68,69]. We return to the effects of statins in more detail in Chapter 4.

As explained earlier in this chapter, all of the major types of vegetable oils consumed in Japan today exhibited diverse toxicity in animal models—inducing stroke, decreasing platelet numbers, causing pathologic changes in the kidney, lung, and brain, causing hypertension, reducing tissue levels of steroid hormones, inducing diabetes mellitus, and/or shortening mean survival time. While the active principles in canola oil have not yet been identified, we do know that two kinds of glucosinolates are converted to many derivatives during absorption and digestion, and that these derivatives exhibit related toxicity [28]. Importantly, these toxic oils exerted survival-shortening activity in a dose-dependent manner in stroke-prone SHRSP rats [75]. Let's also consider the tolerable daily intake (TDI) of canola oil. If we first look at the TDI of polychlorinated biphenyl (PCB, tetra chlorinated form), which exhibited the highest potency found to date to decrease testosterone levels in animal experiments and is now highly regulated, the TDI of PCB (tetra chlorinated form) is 161 pg/kg body weight/day. The estimated intake of the average Japanese is 2.6 pg/kg/day [28], giving an intake/TDI ratio of just <0.02, indicating that regulation of PCB production has successfully reduced the exposure of Japanese people to PCB over time. In the case of canola oil, the TDI has been determined to be 0.033 energy percent of the diet, and the estimated intake of the average Japanese is 5.7 energy percent, giving an intake/TDI ratio of roughly 190 (using survival time of the SHRSP rat as a marker). In the case of canola oil, the active principle has not been identified; therefore, we use energy percent to determine the intake/TDI ratio for canola oil. The ratio for 3-MCPD (monochloropropane-diol) is 1–2.5. Recently, 3-MCPD was found in vegetable oils, and its safety was discussed by the Joint FAO/WHO Expert Committee on Food Additives in 2016 [135]. However, our own reports on the toxicity of canola, olive, and some other vegetable oils (see Chapter 4) have been disregarded by international organizations.

As evidence has accumulated from animal experiments on the mechanisms of vegetable fats and oils, evidence has also accumulated from clinical observational studies and/or interventional studies that high levels of VK2, but not VK1, are inversely associated with cardiovascular mortality, cancer mortality, and lumbar fracture. As predicted, the use of warfarin or dihydro-VK1 resulted in adverse effects [28] (Table 2, p. 25). Thus, the VK2–osteocalcin link is deeply associated with cerebral- and cardiovascular disease, cancer, diabetes mellitus, and chronic kidney disease, as well as mental disorders via the endocrine-disrupting activities of these vegetable fats and oils, and without involving elevated LDL-C levels.

Given the accumulated evidence thus far, we present here the medical hypothesis that increased intake of some vegetable oils and vegetable fats in the presence of roughly comparable amounts of animal fats, as in Japan, is a factor endangering some populations through increasing low birth weight rates, decreasing birth rates, and decreasing populations that are affected by physical and mental disorders.

Supporting lines of evidence in Japan are as follows. (1) The residents of Hisayama Town who closely followed recommendations to increase vegetable oil intake in place of animal fat intake ultimately had a higher prevalence of dementia, higher prevalence of diabetes mellitus, and potentially more stroke events compared with the average Japanese population. (2) The sequence of events that occurred is compatible with a cause-and-effect relationship; that is, the rapid increase in vegetable oil intake between 1965 and 1975 was followed by an increase in diabetes mellitus and kidney disease after around 1980, then by increased rates of low birth weight infants and patients with mental disorders after around 1990, and thereafter by decreasing population levels (Figure 13 and Figures 15, 16, and 25). (3) The known toxic doses of vegetable fats and oils are comparable to the doses ingested by the Japanese population.

3.6. Additional Data Must Be Collected on the Intake of Different Types of Fats and Oils in Different Countries and Ethnic Groups

Both animal experiments and clinical observational studies have shown that higher intakes of cholesterol and animal fats can protect against stroke onset and death from stroke in acutely hospitalized patients. The lifetime risk of stroke is high in East Asia, and in the low-income population in Tianjin, China, stroke (both ischemic and thrombotic) increased 3- to 4-fold between 1992 and 2016, which was correlated with a very high intake ratio of vegetable oil to animal fats (Figures 18 and 19). Stroke morbidity decreased only in Eastern Europe during the same period, which may be explained by the increased intake of animal fats in the region.

We have pointed out that the three countries defeated in the Second World War—Japan, Germany, and Italy—all exhibit highly prevalent dementia (Figure 25, p. 45), changing population pyramids and decreasing populations

(Figure 15, p. 35), and highly prevalent diabetes mellitus [28]. We have not been able to evaluate our medical hypothesis further as there is a definitive lack of intake data for the various types of fats and oils. It is hard to understand why the administrative authorities and industry have not stepped forward to openly disclose exactly which types of vegetable fats and oils are included in our foods.

It is interesting to look at why Japan has a much higher prevalence of cognitive disorders than Korea (24% vs. <10%; Figure 25) in relation to the specialty oil, perilla oil, which is high in ALA. Chinese, Korean, and Japanese cuisine uses various similar ingredients, and while vegetable oils are used abundantly in Chinese dishes, both vegetable oils and animal fats (lard and butter) are widely used in Japanese and Korean dishes. Canola oil is one of the major cooking oils used in Korean cuisine today, so why does South Korea have a lower prevalence of cognitive disorders than Japan? Again, if we look back to earlier in the twentieth century, among victims of the Korean War (1950–1953), it was found that Koreans had less severe vascular conditions than Americans and that this was correlated with larger amounts of α-linolenic acid (ALN, n-3) in plasma lipids. The Korean population is the only population that we know of who continued to produce and consume perilla seeds[6] throughout the Second World War. When animal experiments later demonstrated the safety and usefulness of perilla oil (Table 1, p. 5), the production of perilla seeds began again on a relatively small scale in Japan. Now, the majority of perilla seeds come from northern China, with South Korean imports of perilla seeds at around twice that of Japan, despite Japan's 2-fold greater population. Moreover, Korean people used to consume perilla seed from their fields. So, perilla oil intake in the South Korean population (per capita) is interesting in relation to the relatively low prevalence of cognitive disorders. This finding is also in line with animal experiment findings that, compared with high linoleic safflower oil or soybean oil, perilla oil exhibited anti-aging activity in relation to markers such as survival time, memory and learning ability, and locomotor activity in aging (Table 1, Figure 25).

Chapter 3 Summary

When we look at trends in nutrient intake and disease patterns in Japan over the last several decades, the rapid increase in fat and vegetable oil intake after the Second World War that plateaued around 1975 was accompanied by increased incidence

---

[6] *Perilla frutescens* belongs to genus Lamiaceae as do many herbal plants that are popular in Western countries (e.g., basil, thyme, lavender, and mint). Its origin is said to be the foothills of the Himalayas (relatively cool areas in China, India, and other East Asian countries). In Japan, perilla seeds were traditionally consumed by people living in colder areas by mixing them with many traditional foods, but perilla seed cooking oil stopped being produced as and was replaced with canola and soybean oil before the Second World War.

of lifestyle-related diseases. Similarly, in the Hisayama Study that started in the early 1960s, the strict dietary recommendations to increase the ratios of vegetable oil/animal fats and vegetable protein/animal protein resulted in strikingly increased morbidity from diabetes, stroke, and cognitive disorders among the town's residents.

Although the average life expectancy and healthy life expectancy of Japanese has ranked top globally over the past few decades, the 2017 reports from the UN and OECD alerted us to the reality that Japan and some other countries are experiencing rapid population declines while others are experiencing population increases. In addition to the low birth rate, the Japanese population can be characterized by a high proportion of low birth weight babies and rapid increases in the incidence of mental disorders. We propose that increased intake of vegetable fats and oils with stroke-inducing and endocrine-disrupting activities in countries with restricted intakes of animal fats and cholesterol has led to the critical situation surrounding physical and mental health currently seen in Japan, East Asia, and the Mediterranean countries. A likely mechanism is through inhibition of the VK2–osteocalcin (matrix Gla protein) link by canola oil (glucosinolates), olive oil (?), and dihydro-VK1 in hydrogenated vegetable oils, and increasing numbers of clinical reports consistent with this mechanism support this notion.

4. Comprehensive Risk Management in Japan in Light of the Medical Care Act

In this final chapter, we focus on analyzing the health status of the Japanese population in relation to lifestyle modifications and drug therapy currently in use, and therefore our conclusions may not be applicable to other countries. The clinical reports we cite are mainly from Japan because we know their authors, organizations, and backgrounds relatively well, which helps us to critically evaluate current Japanese guidelines in light of Japan's Medical Care Act.

The principle of medical care is often represented by the Hippocratic oath: "Above all, do no harm" or "First, do no harm". In Japan's Medical Care Act, Chapter 1, Article 1,1,[7] the principle of medical care is explained as follows: "The purpose of this Act is to contribute to the protection of the health of the nation by safeguarding the interests of the *recipients of medical care* and ensuring a system that efficiently delivers good quality and well-suited medical care (truncated)". The position of the *recipients (patients)* is emphasized in Article 1–2 as follows: "Medical care shall be carried out in accordance with the physical and mental state of the *recipient of medical care*, based on a relationship of trust between the physician, dentist, pharmacist, nurse, or other medical care professional and the *recipient of medical care*, in a way which respects life and ensures the dignity of the individual, and shall be of good quality and well-suited (truncated)."

As we were reviewing the relationship between lipid nutrition and diseases, we came to realize that various medical care fields are currently influenced by industry-oriented people legally pursuing interests that are being criticized by those pursuing strictly evidence-based medical care. Also, we found close ties between people in the oil seed industry and those in the livestock and food industry. Hospital management teams and the pharmaceutical, dietary supplement, and food industries all seem to be deeply involved in the recommendations being made for the cholesterol-lowering medications and fats and oils we use. Trying to change this industry-oriented structure will require vast amounts of energy, but recalling the principles of medical care in the Hippocratic Oath and Chapter 1, Article 1 of the Medical Care Act, we need to actively question whether current recommendations in

---

[7] See http://www.japaneselawtranslation.go.jp/law/detail/?id=2199&vm=04&re=02 for the unofficial English translation quoted here, and https://www.mhlw.go.jp/web/t_doc?dataId=80090000&dataType=0&pageNo=1 for the official Japanese original (accessed on 12 January 2021).

the different medical care fields are in fact beneficial for the health of the recipient and the health of the nation.

Historically, global industry has been successful in financially supporting some scientists and giving them a powerful voice in medical societies and medical journals, while also encouraging them to publish guidelines favorable to industry. If medical societies publish guidelines that set very low standard values as "normal" values for health checkups, then the number of patients receiving drug treatment increases, which is favorable to industry. Yet, there are also some medical societies and government-controlled organizations with less relevance to industry that have published much higher standard values, so that the vast number of patients can be free from adverse effects of drugs. Let's look at some cases where Chapter 1 of the Medical Care Act appears not to have been complied with and some cases where it has had a brush with the law.

4.1. Cholesterol-Lowering Medications and the Medical Care Act

Most Japanese people are aware of their blood cholesterol because clinical testing is available at low cost. The test results are stored by different organizations (e.g., at the prefecture, city, and company levels), and several such organizations have analyzed the cholesterol–disease relationship. All of the analyses undertaken have revealed inverse associations between cholesterol level and all-cause mortality, cancer, and cerebrovascular disease, and this is the basis for our conclusion that high cholesterol is a predictor of longevity [10,19]. The so-called "bad cholesterol, good cholesterol hypothesis" has lost all credibility because the LDL-C/HDL-C ratio can be lowered successfully with different drugs but with no benefits observed for all-cause mortality and CHD mortality. Rather, all-cause mortality is increased by such medications.

In the well-known Scandinavian Simvastatin Survival Study (4S Study) published in 1994, simvastatin treatment of patients with CHD aged between 35 and 70 years reduced mortality and morbidity. There was a roughly 30% relative risk reduction in the risk of death, and absolute CHD mortality was reduced from 8.5% to 5.0% [136].

This simvastatin treatment was subsequently applied to Japanese patients with hypercholesterolemia (Japan Lipid Intervention Trial [J-LIT], Figure 27) [137] and the results were published in 2002, 8 years after the 4S Study. Members of the J-LIT Study Group included many important physicians from the Japan Atherosclerosis Society, and yet despite widespread recognition that RCTs produce more reliable results if properly performed, interestingly the effect of simvastatin was reported without a control group in the J-LIT Study (Figure 27).

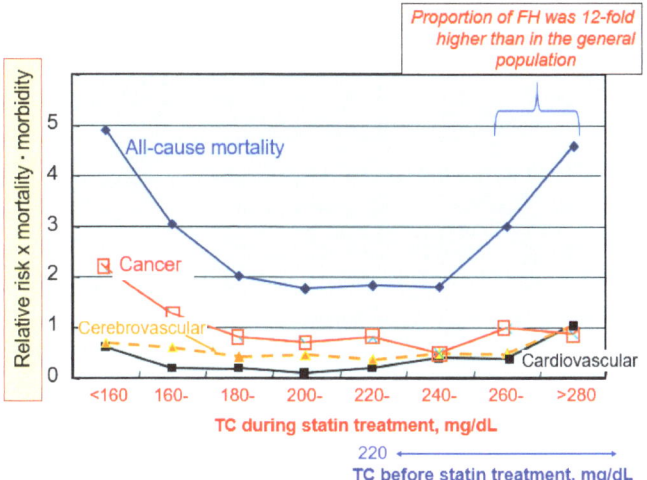

Figure 27. First large-scale intervention trial performed in Japan with low-dose simvastatin. LDL-C during treatment with simvastatin vs. cause-specific morbidity and all-cause mortality. Figure is based on data from Ref. [137]. We have replotted the data so that the relative contribution of different diseases to all-cause mortality is easily visible. See the text for details. FH, familial hypercholesterolemia; TC, total cholesterol.

The cause-specific mortality and morbidity exhibited broad V-shapes, which was inconsistent with what would be expected from the conclusions of the 4S Study even though participants and dose differed between these two simvastatin trials. Curiously, the guidelines from the Japan Atherosclerosis Society set the desirable LDL-C levels (<140 mg/dL) based on CVD only, ignoring the effects of the drug on all other diseases.

The J-LIT participants included a 12-fold higher proportion of people with familial hypercholesterolemia (FH) compared with the general population (0.2%), and these participants with FH are likely to be included in the top two subgroups (Figure 28, p. 54) because they are relatively resistant to statins. In Japan, FH patients are also known to exhibit higher mortality (5-fold higher in heterozygous FH than in the general population [138] compared with the non-FH group. Using these values, we recalculated the contribution of the participants with FH by subtracting them from all participants (Figure 29, p. 55)—the positive association between cholesterol level and CVD mortality disappeared. If we then apply the observations of Mabuchi et al. [138] that CVD mortality in heterozygous FH is 11-fold higher than in the general population, the inverse associations of LDL-C and other diseases would appear as those for many general populations in Japan [10]. We can deduce from this that "the lower, the better hypothesis" is not in fact applicable to the non-FH population.

Needless to say, no statin trials for FH patients have succeeded in reducing CHD mortality in RCTs performed after 2004–2005, when new regulations on clinical trials came into effect [139,140]. Thus, we conclude that the use of cholesterol-lowering medications (with simvastatin as an example here) is not justified.

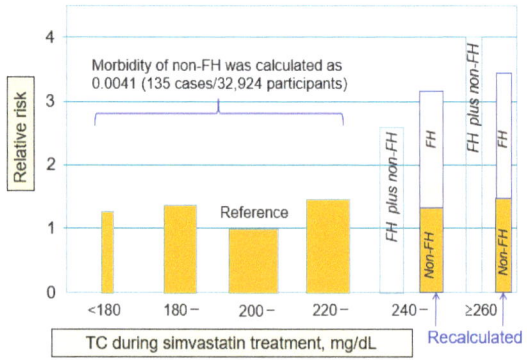

Figure 28. Results of the J-LIT Study with simvastatin were recalculated by separating the FH and non-FH groups, with the following two assumptions: (1) FH cases are located in the two highest LDL-C subgroups during statin treatment, and (2) CHD mortality in FH is 5-fold higher than in the general population. Mabuchi et al. [138] reported 11-fold higher mortality. FH, familial hypercholesterolemia; TC, total cholesterol.

The J-LIT Study was reported as a trial without a control group. However, the findings of the corresponding control study (J-LIT area-controlled follow-up study) were published by different authors in Japanese [141], and one of the interesting conclusions from this control study was that the "dietary advice" given to the control group was the most powerful and the only recognized risk factor for CHD. This dietary advice followed WHO guidelines (i.e., mainstream guidelines). The responsible author of the report was at the top of Japan's National Institute of Health and Nutrition, which publishes "The Dietary Reference Intake for Japanese" every five years; these publications are widely respected by Japanese nutritionists. Instead of changing their recommendations on dietary advice according to their own observations in the "Dietary Reference Intake", they instead adopted the WHO guidelines, which are entirely opposite to the results of their own study. This leaves us questioning the ability of the administrative authorities of Japan to make scientifically sound decisions.

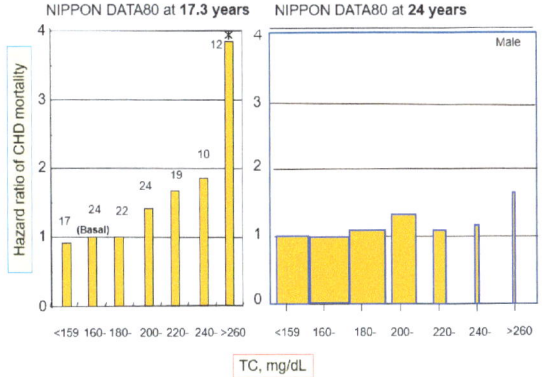

Figure 29. Correlation of ASCVD mortality published by Japan's National Cerebral and Cardiovascular Center. (a) NIPPON DATA80 results published in 2007 for 17.3 years of follow-up [28,142]. Asterisk indicates that only the subgroup with the highest TC value exhibited significantly high CHD mortality. Numbers denote the observed number of cases in each subgroup. (b) NIPPON DATA80 results for 24 years of follow-up [143]. In (b), we have adjusted the column width proportionally to the number of participants in each subgroup. Only the data for males are plotted. CHD, coronary heart disease; TC, total cholesterol.

The findings of a series of follow-up studies performed by the National Cerebrovascular and Cardiovascular Center of Japan, along with the results of the 1980 NIPPON DATA80 study, formed the bases for the guidelines of the Japan Atherosclerotic Society. Our team previously highlighted the insufficient sample size and criticized the associated uncertainty of these studies [19,28]. The results of NIPPON DATA80 at 17.3 years of follow-up (Figure 29a) were apparently consistent with their claim that high cholesterol is a risk for CHD mortality. Recently, however, NIPPON DATA80 findings were published for a longer follow-up period of 24 years and revealed a higher number of deaths (Figure 29b).

Some interesting points can be deduced from Figure 29b where we adjusted the column width proportionally to the number of participants in each subgroup. First, the inverse association of TC with CHD mortality disappeared, and only the subgroup with the highest TC values exhibited high CHD mortality. Among other subgroups with lower TC values, no significant association was found between TC and mortality. This indicates, again, that FH cases must be analyzed separately from the majority of non-FH cases. As no significant correlation was observed among other subgroups, we expected the administrative authorities and medical societies to change their guidelines. Instead of changing them, however, they ignored the 24-year follow-up data for NIPPON DATA80 and adopted the findings of a new smaller-scale study, the Suita Study [144], for their guidelines. Needless to say, the latter study is simply too small to show a clear relationship between cholesterol levels and CVD ($p < 0.02$).

We would like to emphasize that criticizing the Suita Study is not our purpose here; rather we want to press upon the Japan Atherosclerosis Society, associated societies in internal medicine, and members of the administrative authorities (national centers) that revising the guidelines should not be delayed any longer, especially when we have clear evidence that cholesterol-lowering medications afford no beneficial effects for the health of the general population and nation as a whole. They should stop using cholesterol values that give the pharmaceutical industry even more years of sales while, at the same time, the numbers of reports of serious, irreversible adverse effects continue to increase. This is one field of medical care in which the current recommendations related to cholesterol medication and lipid nutrition do not comply with the Medical Care Act.

4.2. Two Different Types of Guidelines for Hypertension, from Different Standpoints of the Medical Care Act

Blood pressure is highly positively associated with ASCVD. Therefore, it is a paradox that hypotensive (anti-hypertensive) drugs, which are effective in lowering blood pressure, fail to reduce stroke mortality and in fact increase it. To try to get to the bottom of this, we carefully reviewed the following four reports on Japanese populations.

1. EPOCH-Japan study involving 39,075 men and women, mean age 60.1 years, followed for 10 years [145]
2. Koriyama Citizen Study involving 14,451 men (mean age 60 ± 10.9 years) and 26,882 women (mean age 62.9 ± 10.1 years), followed for 5.6 years [146]
3. Japan Public Health Center Study involving 15,672 men and women aged 40–69 years, followed for 14 years [103]
4. Ibaraki Prefecture Health Study involving ≥100,000 men and women aged >40 years, followed for 10.5 years [147]

All of these studies reported the failure of hypotensive drugs to lower stroke mortality and instead to increase it strikingly [28]. We view this paradox as a misinterpretation of the causality. The decrease in blood flow due to atherogenesis, inflammation, and/or aging is a critical event and the body raises blood pressure to compensate for it. Thus, hypertension is a marker of both atherogenesis and impaired blood flow, which is rational given the good positive correlations between these two parameters observed in all four reports. The question then is whether hypertension per se stimulates the process of atherogenesis. In inbred strains of rats that develop different degrees of systolic blood pressure—WKY/Kyoto rats (150 mmHg), SHR rats (180 mmHg), and SHRSP rats (250 mmHg)—an atherogenic diet enhanced aortic cholesterol deposition, in reverse order of the blood pressures shown [148]. No clinical data are available to indicate that high blood pressure accelerates aortic cholesterol deposition.

Hypotensive drugs are likely to accelerate the development of ischemic status in the peripheral tissues, increasing stroke incidence, as reported in all four of the abovementioned studies. Peripheral ischemia would increase time spent in bed, as observed in a long-term follow-up study (Figure 30) [149,150]. In all blood pressure subgroups, the proportion of self-dependent people was smaller among users of hypotensive drugs than among non-users.

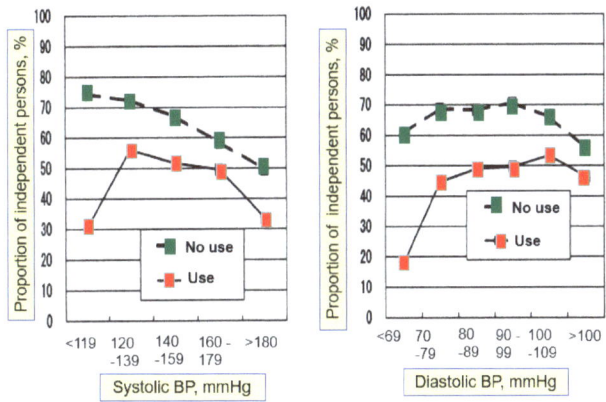

Figure 30. Use of hypotensive drugs decreased the proportion of self-dependent persons over 14 years of follow-up. Figure is based on data from Ref. [149] as analyzed by Hama [150]. Persons who died were not included among the independent persons. BP, blood pressure.

Despite such lines of evidence, those medical organizations with close ties to the pharmaceutical industry, and thus potential COI issues (e.g., the Japan Hypertension Society), keep publishing guidelines with incredibly low standard blood pressure values, even for the elderly population (Table 3, p. 58). However, we are happy to see there are organizations that place greater importance on the scientific evidence available, rather than on economic benefits from associated industries. The government organizations of NICE in the UK and JNC-8 in the USA have notably fewer COI problems compared with the Japan Hypertension Society and the American College of Cardiology/American Heart Association (Table 3).

Table 3. Hypertension guidelines for when to start drug treatment issued by organizations with different degrees of COI issues.

Guidelines Year	COI	Starting Drug Treatment	
NICE, UK 2019 [151]	-	Aged people, 160/100	Those without risk, 160/100
JNC-8, USA 2014 [152]	24% of authors	Age >60 years, 150/90	Age >60 years, 140/90*
Japan Hypertension Society, 2019 [153]	Almost all authors	Age >75 years, 140/90	Age >75 years, 130/80
ACC/AHA, USA, 2017 [154]	Almost all authors	Age >65 years, 130/80	Age >65 years, 130/80

NICE guidelines are from Ref. [151], JNC guidelines are from Ref. [152], Japan Hypertension Society are from Ref. [153], and ACC/AHA guidelines are from Ref. [154]. *Value is presented to avoid confusion across medical fields. Abbreviations: ACC/AHA, American College of Cardiology/American Heart Association; COI, conflict of interest; JNC-8, Eighth Joint National Committee; NICE, National Institute for Health and Care Excellence.

The NICE guidelines do not recommend using hypotensive drugs up to 160/100 mmHg for those without risk [151]. The JNC-8 guidelines state there is no evidence to support beneficial effects of hypotensive drugs for those without risk under 60 years of age, noting that the value presented is to avoid confusion across medical fields [152]. A great many people have blood pressure values between the two standard values (Table 3). As explained above, we cannot find any evidence to support the guidelines issued by the Japan Hypertension Society. Medical care professionals should explain this to patients when obtaining their informed consent, otherwise such medical care could be a violation of the Medical Care Act.

4.3. Failure of Hypoglycemic Medicines to Demonstrate Reductions in All-Cause Mortality in Japan

The number of diabetic patients in Japan increased after around 1980 in line with decreased intake of total energy and carbohydrates and increased intake of vegetable and animal fats and oils (Figure 13, p. 31). We propose that the mechanism underlying this rapid increase in the number of diabetic patients is the inhibition of the VK2–osteocalcin link caused by the increased intake of some kinds of vegetable fats and oils, which in turn impaired functioning of the pancreas, intestines, and other tissues causing insulin resistance (Figure 12, p. 26) [69]. However, across the fields of medical care in Japan, hyperglycemia is taken as the major predictor for the onset of diabetes, and HbA1c (glycosylated hemoglobin) values up to 5.6% are regarded as normal. When health check-up data exceed this level, lifestyle modification is advised, which is effective in the relatively short term in most cases. In the well-controlled

"Look AHEAD Study" [155], intervention comprising rather severe energy restriction and scheduled exercise brought about a 10% decrease in HbA1c within a year, but by 8 years the value had returned to baseline and thereafter increased [156]. During 10 years of this intervention, no significant improvements were observed with respect to CVD death, non-fatal CHD events, non-fatal stroke, or re-hospitalization due to MI. The next step in intervention is using various hypoglycemic drugs to prevent diabetes and its associated fatal diseases.

Often cited are three RCTs that compared standard and intensive therapy groups. In the ACCORD trial [157], median HbA1c levels of 6.4% were achieved in the intensive therapy group at 1 year compared with HbA1c levels of 7.5% in the standard therapy group, but the trial was discontinued after a mean 3.3 years because of increased all-cause and CVD mortality rates. A follow-up study of 1.2 years was added (Accord-ON) [158], but the conclusions were essentially the same [69], despite what we see as some attempts to mislead readers otherwise. In our judgement, the VADT and VADT-On trials [159,160], as well as the ADVANCE and ADVANCE-ON trials [161], reported no promising results of the effectiveness of intensive drug therapy for the prevention of diabetes and associated diseases [69].

Yet, contrary to this evidence, the guidelines of the Japan Diabetes Society as well as those of related societies continue to use a standard HbA1c level of ≤6.5% [162–164].

4.4. Comprehensive Risk Management: The Approach of the Japanese Society of Internal Medicine

ASCVD is positively associated with several factors, and these known risk factors include dyslipidemia (high LDL-C/HDL-C ratio), diabetes, hypertension, and chronic kidney disease. The Japan Atherosclerosis Society published a scheme to figure out the 10-year probability of CHD mortality depending on age, blood pressure, sex, and smoking status, and then treatment goals for LDL-C, HDL-C, and TG (triglyceride) levels are calculated accordingly. We have been critical of this scheme because the calculated treatment goals were not based on scientific evidence [19,28]. In the USA, race and other factors are added, and the 10-year probability of dying of ASCVD can be calculated simply and easily on a pocket calculator without clinicians being involved [165]. An important consideration in risk calculation, diagnosis, and treatment goals for LDL-C is that the causal relationship among these risk factors has not been well clarified or refuted, but still comprehensive risk management is commonly adopted in Japan (Figure 31, p. 60) and possibly in many other countries.

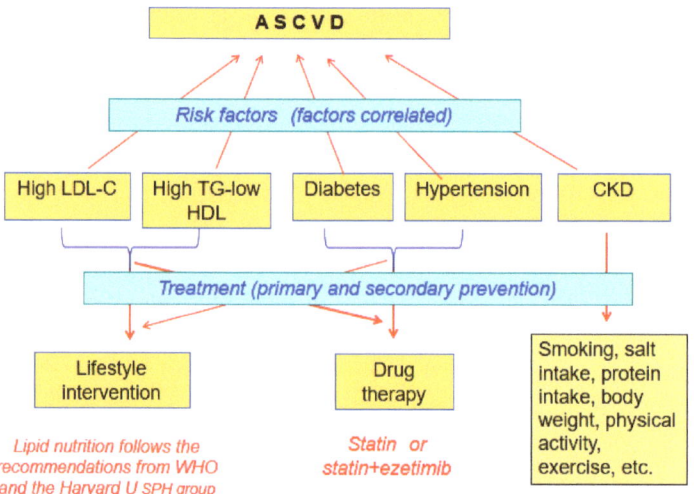

Figure 31. Concept of comprehensive risk management for the prevention of cerebral- and cardiovascular diseases. Shown schematically here based on the Comprehensive Risk Management Chart for Cerebro-Cardiovascular Disease 2019 published by The Japanese Council on Cerebro-Cardiovascular Disease [164]. See the text for details.

In an analysis by the Japanese Society of Internal Medicine, increasing trends in cardiovascular diseases and cardiovascular mortality were found despite successful lowering of blood pressure and smoking rates over the past several decades—we would like to add "and despite extensive use of statins for >30 years" too. Because the national insurance system covers the cost of drugs and health check-ups, Japan's use of statins is probably the highest among industrialized countries.

We point out here the known associated problems: (1) statins cause diabetes to develop, so applying comprehensive risk management as outlined above would increase the chance of pre-diabetic people progressing to ASCVD; (2) cholesterol is necessary for the immunological system to protect against carcinogenesis and infectious diseases, and the chronic use of cholesterol-lowering statins increases all-cause mortality [10,28,166]; (3) statins inhibit the VK2–osteocalcin link leading to kidney lesions and arterial calcification [68,69]; (4) hypotensive drugs accelerate peripheral ischemia resulting in increased ASCVD, particularly stroke; (5) the wrong lipid nutrition is being adopted in lifestyle intervention, based on incorrect recommendations by WHO and the Harvard U SPH group; and (6) statins cause male infertility [167]. Unless these problems are solved, we cannot expect a rapid change in the situation for the declining population of Japan [28].

In 2017, Ueki et al. reported on the latest large-scale RCT performed in Japan, the Japan Diabetes Optimal Integrated Treatment study for three major risk factors of cardiovascular diseases (J-DOIT3) [168]. Intervention was performed to address the three major factors of diabetes, hypertension, and dyslipidemia. This open-label RCT is the most robust clinical trial undertaken in Japan. Conducted at 81 clinical sites, it was led by members of the University of Tokyo Medical School and was supported by government funds as well as by 24 global pharmaceutical companies. The participants were individuals with type 2 diabetes aged 45–69 years who had hypertension, dyslipidemia, or both and were randomly assigned to receive conventional therapy (n=1271) for glucose, blood pressure, and lipid control or intensive therapy (n=1271), which was continued for a median of 8.5 years. The three major risk factors were well controlled, their differences between the two groups were significant ($p = 0.0001$), and the risk factor levels in the intensive therapy group reached the expected levels. However, the most objective endpoint, namely, all-cause death, was essentially the same between the conventional and intensive therapy groups. When publicizing the results, the research group focused on the significant reduction in the hazard ratio for cerebrovascular events (HR = 0.42, $p = 0.002$, rightmost last row of Table 4). However, we do not accept this conclusion because the endpoint, "re-vascularization", was added half way through intervention.

Table 4. Japan Diabetes Optimal Integrated Treatment Study for three major risk factors of cardiovascular diseases.

	Marker			Primary Outcome		Post-Hoc Analysis		
	HbA1c, %	BP, mmHg	LDL-C, mg/dL	MI & stroke event, n	All-cause deaths, n	MI, stroke, revascularization event, n	CHD event, n	Cerebro-vascular event, n
Conventional therapy	7.2	129/74	104	88	48	133	55	42
Intensive therapy	6.8	123/71	85	65	49	109	48	18
Hazard ratio p value	—	— 0.0001	—	0.74 0.055	1.01 0.95	0.81 0.094	0.86 0.44	0.42 0.002

Patients with type 2 diabetes aged 45–69 years with hypertension, dyslipidemia, or both, and an HbA1c of ≥6.9% were randomly assigned (1:1) to receive conventional therapy for glucose, blood pressure, and lipid control (targets: HbA1c <6.9%, blood pressure <130/80 mmHg, LDL cholesterol <120 mg/dL [or 100 mg/dL in patients with a history of coronary artery disease]) or intensive therapy (HbA1c <6.2%, blood pressure <120/75 mm Hg, LDL cholesterol <80 mg/dL in patients with a history of coronary artery disease). Randomization was done using a computer-generated, dynamic balancing method, stratified by sex, age, HbA1c, and history of cardiovascular disease. Neither patients nor investigators were masked to group assignment. The primary outcome was the occurrence of any of a composite of MI, stroke, revascularization (coronary artery bypass surgery, percutaneous transluminal coronary angioplasty, carotid endarterectomy, percutaneous transluminal cerebral angioplasty, and carotid artery stenting), and all-cause mortality. The primary analysis was done in the intention-to-treat population [169]. Abbreviations: CHD, coronary heart disease; BP, blood pressure; LDL-C, low-density lipoprotein cholesterol; MI, myocardial infarction. Important note from us: The data were essentially as reported in the J-DOIT3 study. However, 3 years into the study set with a median intervention of 8.5 years, the number of events was found to be fewer than expected, so "re-vascularization" was newly added as an outcome and the primary and secondary outcome items were rearranged thereafter. Therefore, in this table, we separated the outcomes related to re-vascularization as a post-hoc analysis, simply to avoid confusion [169].

As we were carefully reviewing the results of this study, we encountered serious problems associated with the methodology, scientific rationale, and interpretations. A follow-up study appears to be in progress as described in the Discussion section of the research report, but the intensive therapy used in the J-DOIT3 study is risky in view of currently available evidence, particularly the overly low target HbA1c of 6.2%. We strongly recommend that the J-DOIT3 group inform the participants of the results for the objective endpoints—that there is no difference in mortality—and newly obtain their informed consent following an explanation of the potential risks of the intensive intervention that are now apparent from progress made in this field after the study commenced [169].

In closing, to help demonstrate the problems with current mainstream recommendations in lipid nutrition, we have summarized the differences in nutritional values of different types of fats and oils in Table 5. Although the values were obtained from experimental animal studies, we have included in this book the findings of some clinical observational studies that are consistent with the animal studies, given that RCT trials for many of these parameters are essentially impossible to conduct.

Chapter 4 Summary

In Japan, the general understanding that the nation is healthy has been challenged by a comparison of the country's health status with that in other countries. The results have alerted Japanese medical care professionals to the fact that the nation's health status is, in fact, seriously threatened (as outlined in Chapter 3). We therefore tried to find what mistakes about modifiable factors have been made. In terms of cholesterol-lowering medications, the scientific evidence has been irrationally and incorrectly interpreted. Guidelines for normal blood markers have been irrationally modified by medical societies to favor industry, and drugs to control short- and medium-term biomarkers (e.g., LDL-C, blood pressure, and HbA1c) have failed to achieve the long-term objective endpoint of decreased mortality. Nonetheless, the same medications continue to have adverse effects on patients. It is time for Japanese medical care professionals to ask if the recommended treatments provided comply with the spirit of the Medical Care Act.

Table 5. Safety evaluation of fats and oils in long-term feeding experiments in animal models.

Fats and Oils	Animal or Vegetable	Type of Fats or Oils	Evaluation Based on Animal Experiment
Fats	Animal	Butter, lard, beef tallow	Suppressive for stroke onset, and recommended that average levels be increased to those of the UK and USA
	Vegetable	Palm oil, coconut oil, palm kernel oil	Stroke-inducing and endocrine-disrupting activity reported. Safety not established.
	Hydrogenated vegetable oil	Hydrogenated canola oil, hydrogenated soybean oil	Not suitable for human use due to dihydro-VK1
Oils	Animal	Fish oil (EPA-rich type), fish oil (DHA-rich type)	Prevention of cerebro- and cardiovascular disease and anti-inflammatory effects expected
	Vegetable	Rapeseed oil (canola type, erucic acid-rich type)	Not suitable for human use, due to strong stroke-inducing and endocrine-disrupting activity
		Soybean oil (linoleic-rich type), safflower oil (linoleic-rich type), rice bran oil, sesame oil, sunflower oil (linoleic-rich type)	Care needed to avoid excessive intake as n-6/n-3 ratios are high
		Olive oil, sunflower oil (oleic-rich type), safflower oil (oleic-rich type)	Not suitable for human use due to activity that induces stroke and shortens survival
		Soybean oil (oleic-rich type)	No convincing safety evidence available
		Perilla oil, linseed oil	Highly safe, and recommend for cooking in place of common cooking oils
	Microbial fermentation product	Linolenic-rich oil (n-6)	Not recommended for human use because it increases arachidonic acid
		Arachidonic acid-rich oil ($\omega 6$)	Not suitable for human use because of teratogenicity problem
		DHA-rich oil ($\omega 3$)	Safety evaluation required

Epilogue

Industry-oriented scientists developed an apparently rational means to convince people that drug treatment is clinically effective—*the systematic survey of RCT reports and meta-analysis of their reported results*. However, the drawbacks of this method are as follows.

(1) It is not easy for readers to re-examine the validity of the data, which typically include a huge number of subjects. Also, if even a small amount of unpublished data make their way into a meta-analysis, this allows for conclusions to be easily modified, as happened in the Oxford PSC (Prospective Studies Collaboration) and CTSU (Clinical Trial Service Unit & Epidemiologic) studies [170], the associated problems for which we have previously critically reviewed [171].

(2) Global industry has successfully increased the number of industry-oriented scientists who are influential in medical societies with journals that can publish their articles, and this has led to increased numbers of industry-oriented articles being published (publication bias).

(3) Not all published articles are of the same quality and aside from the issue of potentially including some questionable data, some articles may even include intentional misrepresentations designed to deceive naive readers [172,173].

Thus, we should be wary of relying solely on the findings of current meta-analyses to determine the basis of our recommendations, unless we can find a better way to avoid scientifically incorrect or questionable data from being included in the large datasets used.

Despite the major scientific basis for cholesterol-lowering medication having lost credibility, industry-oriented people have found different ways to maintain the status quo; for example, by including non-objective endpoints such as non-fatal MI events, non-fatal stroke events, and re-hospitalization. On the one hand, we feel we should accept the diagnosis of the doctor in charge as long as the decision to use or not use statins is readily clear, but on the other hand, looking back at the development of statins, clinical reports on their efficacy and adverse effects, and the many conflicting issues that appeared, we cannot accept using such non-objective endpoints to justify their continued recommended use. Industry-oriented people should demonstrate that statins can in fact reduce objective measures such as MI mortality, ASCVD mortality, or all-cause mortality. While the early 21st century may be a time of close ties between global industry and the administrative authorities, the general public is left largely unaware of the many important issues we have raised here, which directly impact their health and longevity.

Key Issues

In current medical practice for the prevention of ASCVD, risk factors such as high blood cholesterol, hypertension, hyperglycemia (diabetes), and chronic kidney disease are interpreted to be causative, and their comprehensive management is considered the "royal road" to preventing lifestyle-related diseases. However, their causal relationships have not been established, and drug therapy to control these short- and medium-term biomarkers (risk factors) has not been successful in achieving the goal of reduced all-cause mortality. Instead, based on the pharmacological mechanisms revealed mainly by animal experiments and the findings of clinical studies consistent with these mechanisms, we have proposed that some types of vegetable fats and oils exhibit stroke-inducing and endocrine-disrupting activity and that their inhibition of the vitamin K2–osteocalcin link is the major cause of ASCVD and related diseases. Clinical reports consistent with this proposed mechanism continue to accumulate. We are concerned that medical care professionals continue to insist on the current approach, which will only heighten the disastrous health problems that Japan and some countries are facing. Many aspects of our current medical practice in Japan are likely to be in conflict with the Medical Care Act.

Notes Added in Proof

1. Recently, both high-oleic and high-linoleic soybean oils were reported to up-regulate the oxytocin genes in the hypothalamus and raise plasma oxytocin levels in mice [174]. This endocrine-disrupting activity appears to be different from that we observed in the SHRSP rat (Figure 21, p. 41), although high-oleic soybean oil has not been available for us to assess its safety.

2. Guasch-Ferré et al. recently reported that the substitution of margarine, butter, mayonnaise, and dairy fat with olive oil could lead to lower risks of CHD and CVD [175], which is entirely inconsistent with our recommendations in this book. We have critically reviewed reports from the Harvard U SPH group [6–8], but our criticisms [28 and this book] apply to this new report mostly from the same group [175].

3. In Japan, The Japanese Society of Hypertension Guidelines for the Management of Hypertension (JSH 2019) have been published. Like the JSH, we share the understanding that blood pressure is positively associated with many types of lifestyle-related diseases, and that lowering blood pressure by changing diet and increasing physical activity would be the likely means for prevention, although we take the opposite view on dietary means with respect to the choice of vegetable oils and animal fats. Moreover, we and the JSH group came to opposite conclusions on the effectiveness of hypotensive drugs when long-term consequences (mortality from cardio- and cerebrovascular diseases and the proportion of the population living independently) were the endpoints. Despite the vast amount of survey data available and involvement of many specialists in hypertension, the evidence in the JSH 2019 fails to demonstrate that these parameters were actually lowered by hypotensive drugs. We retain the conclusions described in Chapter 4.2. that hypotensive drugs are likely to elevate these parameters by reducing blood flow and impairing peripheral tissue functioning due to vegetable oil toxicity.

Supplementary Materials: Figure S1: Fatty acid composition of animal & vegetable fats and oils.

Funding: Kinjo Gakuin University Research Grant; in part by scholarship donations to Kinjo Gakuin University from Sugiyama Drug Co., Ltd. and Ohta Oil Co., Ltd.; a research grant from Nagoya City; and governmental grants from the Ministry of Health, Labour and Welfare and the Ministry of Education, Culture, Sports, Science and Technology, Japan.

Conflicts of Interest: The authors declared no conflicts of interest, based on the guidelines of the Japan Society for Lipid Nutrition (J Lipid Nutrition 2919; 28:62-66).

References

1. Keys, A.; Anderson, J.T.; Grande, F. Serum cholesterol response to changes in the diet: IV. Particular saturated fatty acids in the diet. *Metabolism* **1965**, *14*, 776–787. [CrossRef]
2. Hegsted, D.M.; McGandy, R.B.; Myers, M.L.; Stare, F.J. Quantitative effects of dietary fat on serum cholesterol in man. *Am. J. Clin. Nutr.* **1965**, *17*, 281–295. [CrossRef]
3. Derr, J.; Kris-Etherton, P.M.; Pearson, T.A.; Seligson, F.H. The role of fatty acid saturation on plasma lipids, lipoproteins, and apolipoproteins: II. The plasma total and low-density lipoprotein cholesterol response of individual fatty acids. *Metabolism* **1993**, *42*, 130–134. [CrossRef]
4. Multiple Risk Factor Intervention Trial Research Group. Multiple risk factor intervention trial: Risk factor changes and mortality results. *JAMA* **1982**, *248*, 1465–1477. [CrossRef]
5. Strandberg, T.E.; Salomaa, V.V.; Naukkarinen, V.A.; Vanhanen, H.T.; Sarna, S.J.; Miettinen, T.A. Long-term mortality after 5-year multifactorial primary prevention of cardiovascular diseases in middle-aged men. *JAMA* **1991**, *266*, 1225–1229. [CrossRef] [PubMed]
6. Ascherio, A.; Rimm, E.B.; Giovannucci, E.L.; Spiegelman, D.; Stampfer, M.; Willet, W.C. Dietary fat and risk of coronary heart disease in men: cohort follow up study in the United States. *BMJ* **1996**, *313*, 84–90. [CrossRef]
7. Hu, F.B.; Stampfer, M.J.; Manson, J.E.; Ascherio, A.; Colditz, G.A.; Speizer, F.E.; Hennekens, C.H.; Willet, W.C. Dietary saturated fats and their food sources in relation to the risk of coronary heart disease in women. *Am. J. Clin. Nutr.* **1999**, *70*, 1001–1008. [CrossRef]
8. Mozaffarian, D.; Katan, M.B.; Ascherio, A.; Stampfer, M.J.; Willet, W.C. Trans-fatty acids and cardiovascular disease. *N. Engl. J. Med.* **2006**, *354*, 1601–1613. [CrossRef] [PubMed]
9. Wang, Q.; Afshin, A.; Yakoob, M.Y.; Singh, G.M.; Rehm, C.D.; Khatibzadeh, S.; Micha, R.; Shi, P.; Mozaffarian, D.; Global Burden of Diseases Nutrition and Chronic Diseases Expert Group (NutriCoDE). Impact of nonoptimal intakes of saturated, polyunsaturated, and trans-fat on global burdens of coronary heart disease. *J. Am. Heart Assoc.* **2016**, *5*, e002891. [CrossRef]
10. Okuyama, H.; Ichikawa, Y.; Sun, Y.J.; Hamazaki, T.; Lands, W.E.M. *Prevention of Coronary Heart Disease: From the Cholesterol Hypothesis to ω6 to ω3 Balance*; Karger: Basel, Switzerland, 2007.
11. Strandberg, T.E.; Salomaa, V.V.; Vanhanen, H.T.; Naukkarinen, V.A.; Sarna, S.J.; Miettinen, T.A. Mortality in participants and non-participants of a multifactorial prevention study of cardiovascular diseases: A 28 year follow up of the Helsinki Businessmen Study. *Br. Heart J.* **1995**, *74*, 449–454. [CrossRef] [PubMed]

12. Ramsden, C.E.; Zamora, D.; Leelarthaepin, B.; Majchrzak-Hong, S.F.; Faurot, K.R.; Suchindran, C.M.; Ringel, A.; Davis, J.M.; Hibbeln, J.R. Use of dietary linoleic acid for secondary prevention of coronary heart disease and death: Evaluation of recovered data from the Sydney Diet Heart Study and updated meta-analysis. *BMJ* **2013**, *346*, e8707. [CrossRef] [PubMed]
13. Ramsden, C.E.; Zamora, D.; Majchrzak-Hong, S.; Faurot, K.R.; Broste, S.K.; Frantz, R.P.; Davis, J.M.; Ringel, A.; Suchindran, C.M.; Hibbeln, J.R. Re-evaluation of the traditional diet-heart hypothesis: analysis of recovered data from Minnesota Coronary Experiment (1968-73). *BMJ* **2016**, *353*, i1246. [CrossRef] [PubMed]
14. Muldoon, M.F.; Manuck, S.B.; Matthews, K.A. Lowering cholesterol concentrations and mortality: a quantitative review of primary prevention trials. *BMJ* **1990**, *301*, 309–314. [CrossRef]
15. Harcombe, Z.; Baker, J.S.; Cooper, S.M.; Davies, B.; Sculthorpe, N.; DiNicolantonio, J.J.; Grace, F. Evidence from randomized controlled trials did not support the introduction of dietary fat guidelines in 1977 and 1983: A systematic review and meta-analysis. *Open Heart* **2015**, *2*, e000196. [CrossRef] [PubMed]
16. Ravnskov, U. *Fat and Cholesterol Are Good for You*; GB Publishing Ltd.: Merseyside, UK, 2009.
17. Turpeinen, O.; Karvonen, M.J.; Pekkarinen, M.; Miettinen, M.; Elosuo, R.; Paavilainen, E. Dietary prevention of coronary heart disease: the Finnish Mental Hospital Study. *Int. J. Epidemiol.* **1979**, *8*, 99–118. [CrossRef] [PubMed]
18. Teicholz, N.; Thorn, E. Saturated Fats and CVD: AHA Convicts, We Say Acquit. *Medscape*. 12 July 2017. Available online: https://www.medscape.com/viewarticle/882564 (accessed on 18 August 2020).
19. Hamazaki, T.; Okuyama, H.; Ogushi, Y.; Hama, R. Towards a paradigm shift in cholesterol treatment. A re-examination of the cholesterol issue in Japan. *Ann. Nutr. Metab.* **2015**, *66* (Suppl. 4), 1–116. [PubMed]
20. Shimokawa, T.; Horiuchi, A.; Hori, T.; Saito, M.; Naito, Y.; Kabasawa, H.; Nagae, Y.; Matsubara, M.; Okuyama, H. Effect of dietary alpha-linolenate/linoleate balance on mean survival time, incidence of stroke and blood pressure of spontaneously hypertensive rats. *Life Sci.* **1988**, *43*, 2067–2075. [CrossRef]
21. Okuyama, H.; Langsjoen, P.H.; Langsjoen, A.M.; Ohara, N. Industrial control of guidelines for lipid nutrition. In *Fat and Cholesterol Don't Cause Heart Attacks and Statins Are Not the Solution*; Rosch, P.J., Ed.; Columbus Publishing Ltd.: Cwmbran, UK, 2016; pp. 73–112.
22. Dyerberg, J.; Bang, H.O.; Stoffersen, E.; Moncada, S.; Vane, J.R. Eicosapentaenoic acid and prevention of thrombosis and atherosclerosis? *Lancet* **1978**, *2*, 117–119. [CrossRef]
23. Kita, Y.; Shindou, H.; Shimizu, T. Cytosolic phospholipase A 2 and lysophospholipid acyltransferases. *Biochim. Biophys. Acta Mol. Cell Biol. Lipids* **2019**, *1864*, 838–845. [CrossRef]
24. Aoki, J. Mechanisms of lysophosphatidic acid production. *Semin. Cell Dev. Biol.* **2004**, *15*, 477–489. [CrossRef]

25. Matsuda, S.; Inoue, T.; Lee, H.-C.; Kono, N.; Tanaka, F.; Gengyo-Ando, K.; Mitani, S.; Arai, H. Member of the membrane-bound O-acyltransferase (MBOAT) family encodes a lysophospholipid acyltransferase with broad substrate specificity. *Genes Cells* **2008**, *13*, 879–888. [CrossRef]
26. Bibus, D.; Lands, B. Balancing proportions of competing omega-3 and omega-6 highly unsaturated fatty acids (HUFA) in tissue lipids. *Prostaglandins Leukot. Essent. Fatty Acids* **2015**, *99*, 19–23. [CrossRef]
27. Walker, C.G.; West, A.L.; Browning, L.M.; Madden, J.; Gambel, J.M.; Jebb, S.A.; Calder, P.C. The pattern of fatty acids displaced by EPA and DHA following 12 months supplementation varies between blood cell and plasma fractions. *Nutrients* **2015**, *7*, 6281–6893. [CrossRef]
28. Okuyama, H.; Ohara, N.; Kobayashi, T.; Hama, R.; Uchino, H.; Iwamoto, T.; Hashimoto, M.; Kagohashi, Y.; Watanabe, S.; Sakai, K.; et al. *Is the Wrong Kind of Lipid Nutrition Endangering the Japanese People?* Sefof Council Japan & Chunichi Publishing Ltd.: Nagoya, Japan, 2019. (In Japanese)
29. Lands, W.E.M. *Fish, Omega-3 and Human Health*, 2nd ed.; AOCS Publishing: Urbana, IL, USA, 2005.
30. Smith, W.L.; DeWitt, D.L.; Garavito, R.M. Cyclooxygenases: structural, cellular, and molecular biology. *Annu. Rev. Biochem.* **2000**, *69*, 145–82. [CrossRef]
31. Smith, W.L. Cyclooxygenases, peroxide tone and the allure of fish oil. *Curr. Opin. Cell Biol.* **2005**, *17*, 174–182. [CrossRef] [PubMed]
32. Wada, M.; DeLong, C.J.; Hong, Y.H.; Rieke, C.J.; Song, I.; Sidhu, R.S.; Yuan, C.; Warnock, M.; Schmaier, A.H.; Yokoyama, C.; et al. Enzymes and receptors of prostaglandin pathways with arachidonic acid-derived versus eicosapentaenoic acid-derived substrates and products. *J. Biol. Chem.* **2007**, *282*, 22254–22266. [CrossRef] [PubMed]
33. Hammarström, S. Leukotriene C5: a slow reacting substance derived from eicosapentaenoic acid. *J. Biol. Chem.* **1980**, *255*, 7093–7094. [CrossRef]
34. Leitch, A.G.; Lee, T.H.; Ringel, E.W.; Prickett, J.D.; Robinson, D.R.; Pyne, S.G.; Corey, E.J.; Drazen, J.M.; Austen, K.F.; Lewis, R.A. Immunologically induced generation of tetraene and pentaene leukotrienes in the peritoneal cavities of menhaden-fed rats. *J. Immunol.* **1984**, *132*, 2559–2265. [PubMed]
35. Wallace, J.L.; McKnight, G.W. Comparison of the damage-promoting effects of leukotrienes derived from eicosapentaenoic acid and arachidonic acid on the rat stomach. *J. Exp. Med.* **1990**, *171*, 1827–1832. [CrossRef]
36. Yamamoto, N.; Saitoh, M.; Moriuchi, A.; Nomura, M.; Okuyama, H. Effect of dietary alpha-linolenate/linoleate balance on brain lipid compositions and learning ability of rats. *J. Lipid. Res.* **1987**, *28*, 144–151. [CrossRef]
37. Okaniwa, Y.; Yuasa, S.; Yamamoto, N.; Watanabe, S.; Kobayashi, T.; Okuyama, H.; Nomura, M.; Nagata, Y. High linoleate and a high alpha-linolenate diet induced changes in learning behavior of rats. Effects of a shift in diets and reversal of training stimuli. *Biol. Pharm. Bull.* **1996**, *19*, 536–540. [CrossRef]

38. Carlson, S.E.; Colombo, J. Docosahexaenoic acid and arachidonic acid nutrition in early development. *Adv. Pediatr.* **2016**, *63*, 453–471. [CrossRef] [PubMed]
39. Huan, M.; Hamazaki, K.; Sun, Y.; Itomura, M.; Liu, H.; Kang, W.; Watanabe, S.; Terasawa, K.; Hamazaki, T. Suicide attempt and n-3 fatty acid levels in red blood cells: a case control study in China. *Biol. Psychiatry* **2004**, *56*, 490–496. [CrossRef] [PubMed]
40. Hibbeln, J.R. From homicide to happiness–a commentary on omega-3 fatty acids in human society. *Nutr. Health* **2007**, *19*, 9–19. [CrossRef]
41. Okuyama, H.; Kobayashi, T.; Watanabe, S. Dietary fatty acids–the N-6/N-3 balance and chronic elderly diseases. Excess linoleic acid and relative N-3 deficiency syndrome seen in Japan. *Prog. Lipid Res.* **1996**, *35*, 409–457. [CrossRef]
42. Matsuba, S.; Itoh, M.; Joh, T.; Takeyama, H.; Dohi, N.; Watanabe, S.; Okuyama, H. Effect of dietary linoleate/alpha-linolenate balance on experimentally induced gastric injury in rats. *Prostaglandins Leukot. Essent. Fatty Acids* **1998**, *59*, 317–323. [CrossRef]
43. Serhan, C.N. Pro-resolving lipid mediators are leads for resolution physiology. *Nature* **2014**, *510*, 92–101. [CrossRef] [PubMed]
44. Miyata, J.; Arita, M. Role of omega-3 fatty acids and their metabolites in asthma and allergic diseases. *Allergol. Int.* **2015**, *64*, 27–34. [CrossRef]
45. Asatryan, A.; Bazan, N.G. Molecular mechanisms of signaling via the docosanoid neuroprotectin D1 for cellular homeostasis and neuroprotection. *J. Biol. Chem.* **2017**, *292*, 12390–12397. [CrossRef]
46. Calder, P.C. Very long-chain n-3 fatty acids and human health: fact, fiction and the future. *Proc. Nutr. Soc.* **2018**, *77*, 52–72. [CrossRef]
47. Kroman, N.; Green, A. Epidemiological studies in the Upernavik district, Greenland. Incidence of some chronic diseases 1950-1974. *Acta Med. Scand.* **1980**, *208*, 401–406. [CrossRef]
48. Simopoulos, A.P.; Koletzko, B.; Anderson, R.E.; Hornstra, G.; Mensink, R.P.; Weksler, B.B.; Harris, W.S.; De Caterina, R.; Muggli, R.; Sprecher, H. The 1st Congress of the International Society for the Study of Fatty Acids and Lipids (ISSFAL): fatty acids and lipids from cell biology to human disease. *J. Lipid. Res.* **1994**, *35*, 169–173. [CrossRef]
49. Hirauchi, K.; Sakano, T.; Notsumoto, S.; Nagaoka, T.; Morimoto, A.; Fujimoto, K.; Masuda, S.; Suzuki, Y. Measurement of K vitamins in animal tissues by high-performance liquid chromatography with fluorometric detection. *J. Chromatogr.* **1989**, *497*, 131–137. [CrossRef]
50. Kamao, M.; Suhara, Y.; Tsugawa, N.; Uwano, M.; Yamaguchi, N.; Uenishi, K.; Ishida, H.; Sasaki, S.; Okano, T. Vitamin K content of foods and dietary vitamin K intake in Japanese young women. *J. Nutr. Sci. Vitaminol. (Tokyo)* **2007**, *53*, 464–470. [CrossRef]
51. Demopoulos, C.A.; Pinckard, R.N.; Hanahan, D.J. Platelet-activating factor. Evidence for 1-O-alkyl-2-acetyl-sn-glyceryl-3-phosphorylcholine as the active component (a new class of lipid chemical mediators). *J. Biol. Chem.* **1979**, *254*, 355–358. [CrossRef]

52. Horii, T.; Satouchi, K.; Kobayashi, Y.; Saito, K.; Watanabe, S.; Yoshida, Y.; Okuyama, H. Effect of dietary alpha-linolenate on platelet-activating factor production in rat peritoneal polymorphonuclear leukocytes. *J. Immunol.* **1991**, *147*, 1607–1613. [PubMed]
53. Oh-hashi, K.; Takahashi, T.; Watanabe, S.; Kobayashi, T.; Okuyama, H. Possible mechanisms for the differential effects of high linoleate safflower oil and high alpha-linolenate perilla oil diets on platelet-activating factor production by rat polymorphonuclear leukocytes. *J. Lipid Mediat. Cell Signal.* **1997**, *17*, 207–220. [CrossRef]
54. Devane, W.A.; Hanus, L.; Breuer, A.; Pertwee, R.G.; Stevenson, L.A.; Griffin, G.; Gibson, D.; Mandelbaum, A.; Etinger, A.; Mechoulam, R. Isolation and structure of a brain constituent that binds to the cannabinoid receptor. *Science* **1992**, *258*, 1946–1949. [CrossRef]
55. Mechoulam, R.; Fride, E. The unpaved road to the endogenous brain cannabinoid ligands, the anandamides. In *Cannabinoid Receptors*; Pertwee, R.G., Ed.; Academic Press: Boston, MA, USA, 1995; pp. 233–258.
56. Sugiura, T.; Kondo, S.; Kishimoto, S.; Miyashita, T.; Nakane, S.; Kodaka, T.; Suhara, Y.; Takayama, H.; Waku, K. Evidence that 2-arachidonoylglycerol but not N-palmitoylethanolamine or anandamide is the physiological ligand for the cannabinoid CB2 receptor. Comparison of the agonistic activities of various cannabinoid receptor ligands in HL-60 cells. *J. Biol. Chem.* **2000**, *275*, 605–612. [CrossRef] [PubMed]
57. Kang, J.X. A transgenic mouse model for gene-nutrient interactions. *J. Nutrigenet. Nutrigenomics* **2008**, *1*, 172–177. [CrossRef]
58. Kang, J.X.; Gleason, E.D. Omega-3 fatty acids and hippocampal neurogenesis in depression. *CNS Neurol. Disord. Drug Targets* **2013**, *12*, 460–465. [CrossRef]
59. Abdelhamid, A.S.; Brown, T.J.; Brainard, J.S.; Biswas, P.; Thorpe, G.C.; Moore, H.J.; Deane, K.H.; AlAbdulghafoor, F.K.; Summerbell, C.D.; Worthington, H.V.; et al. Omega-3 fatty acids for the primary and secondary prevention of cardiovascular disease. *Cochrane Database Syst. Rev.* **2018**, *11*, CD003177. [CrossRef]
60. Hirai, A.; Hamazaki, T.; Terano, T.; Nishikawa, T.; Tamura, Y.; Kumagai, A.; Sajiki, J. Eicosapentaenoic acid and platelet function in Japanese. *Lancet* **1980**, *316*, 1132–1133. [CrossRef]
61. Terano, T.; Hirai, A.; Hamazaki, T.; Kobayashi, S.; Fujita, T.; Tamura, Y.; Kumagai, A. Effect of oral administration of highly purified eicosapentaenoic acid on platelet function, blood viscosity and red cell deformability in healthy human subjects. *Atherosclerosis* **1983**, *46*, 321–231. [CrossRef]
62. Hamazaki, T.; Hirai, A.; Terano, T.; Sajiki, J.; Kondo, S.; Fujita, T.; Tamura, Y.; Kumagai, A. Effects of orally administered ethyl ester of eicosapentaenoic acid (EPA; C20:5, omega-3) on PGI2-like substance production by rat aorta. *Prostaglandins* **1982**, *23*, 557–567. [CrossRef]
63. Hirai, A.; Terano, T.; Hamazaki, T.; Sajiki, J.; Kondo, S.; Ozawa, A.; Fujita, T.; Miyamoto, T.; Tamura, Y.; Kumagai, A. The effects of the oral administration of fish oil concentrate on the release and the metabolism of [14C]arachidonic acid and [14C]eicosapentaenoic acid by human platelets. *Thromb. Res.* **1982**, *28*, 285–298. [CrossRef]
64. Kobayashi, S.; Hirai, A.; Terano, T.; Hamazaki, T.; Tamura, Y.; Kumagai, A. Reduction in blood viscosity by eicosapentaenoic acid. *Lancet* **1981**, *2*, 197. [CrossRef]

65. Nagata, M.; Hata, J.; Hirakawa, Y.; Mukai, N.; Yoshida, D.; Ohara, T.; Kishimoto, H.; Kawano, H.; Kitazono, T.; Kiyohara, T.; Ninomiya, T. The ratio of serum eicosapentaenoic acid to arachidonic acid and risk of cancer death in a Japanese community: The Hisayama Study. *J. Epidemiol.* **2017**, *27*, 578–583. [CrossRef]
66. Sekikawa, A.; Curb, J.D.; Ueshima, H.; El-Saed, A.; Kadowaki, T.; Abbott, R.D.; Evans, R.W.; Beatriz, L.R.; Okamura, T.; Sutton-Tyrrell, K.; et al. Marine-derived n-3 fatty acids and atherosclerosis in Japanese, Japanese-American, and Whites: a cross-sectional study. *J. Am. Coll. Cardiol.* **2008**, *52*, 417–424. [CrossRef]
67. Sacks, F.M.; Lichtenstein, A.H.; Wu, J.H.Y.; Appel, L.J.; Creager, M.A.; Kris-Etherton, P.M.; Miller, M.; Rimm, E.B.; Rudel, L.L.; Robinson, J.G.; et al. Dietary fats and cardiovascular disease: a presidential advisory from the American Heart Association. *Circulation* **2017**, *136*, e1–e23. [CrossRef]
68. Okuyama, H.; Langsjoen, P.H.; Hamazaki, T.; Ogushi, Y.; Hama, R.; Kobayashi, T.; Uchino, H. Statins stimulate atherosclerosis and heart failure: pharmacological mechanisms. *Expert Rev. Clin. Pharmacol.* **2015**, *8*, 189–199. [CrossRef]
69. Okuyama, H.; Langsjoen, P.H.; Ohara, N.; Hashimoto, Y.; Hamazaki, T.; Yoshida, S.; Kobayashi, T.; Langsjoen, A.M. Medicines and vegetable oils as hidden causes of cardiovascular disease and diabetes. *Pharmacology* **2016**, *98*, 134–170. [CrossRef]
70. Prospective Urban Rural Epidemiology (PURE) Study Investigators; Dehghan, M.; Mente, A.; Zhang, X.; Swaminathan, S.; Li, W.; Mohan, V.; Iqbal, R.; Kumar, R.; Wentzel-Viljoen, E.; Rosengren, A.; et al. Associations of fats and carbohydrate intake with cardiovascular disease and mortality in 18 countries from five continents (PURE): a prospective cohort study. *Lancet* **2017**, *390*, 2050–2062. [CrossRef]
71. Shibata, H. *Malnutrition in Japan Threatens Longevity. Food Intake and Long Life*; LAP Lambert Academic Publishing: Saarbrücken, Germany, 2018.
72. Okamoto, K.; Aoki, K. Development of a strain of spontaneously hypertensive rats. *Jpn. Circ. J.* **1963**, *27*, 282–293. [CrossRef]
73. Yamori, Y. Implication of hypertensive rat models for primordial nutritional prevention of cardiovascular diseases. *Clin. Exp. Pharmacol. Physiol.* **1999**, *26*, 568–572. [CrossRef]
74. Aoki, K.; Yamori, Y.; Ooshima, A.; Okamoto, K. Effects of high or low sodium intake in spontaneously hypertensive rats. *Jpn. Circ. J.* **1972**, *36*, 539–545. [CrossRef]
75. Huang, M.Z.; Naito, Y.; Watanabe, S.; Kobayashi, T.; Kanai, H.; Nagai, H.; Okuyama, H. Effect of rapeseed and dietary oils on the mean survival time of stroke-prone spontaneously hypertensive rats. *Biol. Pharm. Bull.* **1996**, *19*, 554–557. [CrossRef] [PubMed]
76. Ratnayake, W.M.; Plouffe, L.; Hollywood, R.; L'Abbé, M.R.; Hidiroglou, N.; Sarwar, G.; Mueller, R. Influence of sources of dietary oils on the life span of stroke-prone spontaneously hypertensive rats. *Lipids* **2000**, *35*, 409–420. [CrossRef]
77. Ratnayake, W.M.; L'Abbé, M.R.; Mueller, R.; Hayward, S.; Plouffe, L.; Hollywood, R.; Trick, K. Vegetable oils high in phytosterols make erythrocytes less deformable and shorten the life span of stroke-prone spontaneously hypertensive rats. *J. Nutr.* **2000**, *130*, 1166–1178. [CrossRef]

78. Ogawa, H.; Yamamoto, K.; Kamisako, T.; Meguro, T. Phytosterol additives increase blood pressure and promote stroke onset in salt-loaded stroke-prone spontaneously hypertensive rats. *Clin. Exp. Pharmacol. Physiol.* **2003**, *30*, 919–924. [CrossRef] [PubMed]
79. Tatematsu, K.; Fuma, S.Y.; Satoh, J.; Ichikawa, Y.; Fujii, Y.; Okuyama, H. Dietary canola and soybean oil fed to SHRSP rat dams differently affect the growth and survival of their male pups. *J. Nutr.* **2004**, *134*, 1347–1352. [CrossRef]
80. Innis, S.M.; Dyer, R.; Wadsworth, L.; Quinlan, P.; Diersen-Schade, D. Dietary saturated, monounsaturated, n-6 and n-3 fatty acids, and cholesterol influence platelet fatty acids in the exclusively formula-fed piglet. *Lipids* **1993**, *28*, 645–650. [CrossRef]
81. Miyazawa, D.; Ohara, N.; Yamada, K.; Yasui, Y.; Kitamori, K.; Saito, Y.; Usumi, K.; Nagata, T.; Nonogaki, T.; Hashimoto, Y.; et al. Dietary soybean oil, canola oil and partially-hydrogenated soybean oil affect testicular tissue and steroid hormone levels differently in the miniature pig. *Food Chem. Toxicol.* **2020**, *135*, 110927. [CrossRef] [PubMed]
82. Rotkiewicz, T.; Bomba, G.; Falkowski, J.; Glogowski, J.; Kozera, W.; Kozłowski, M. Studies on a long-term use of rapeseed products in diets for boars. Pathomorphological changes in the reproductive system, liver and thyroid gland. *Reprod. Nutr. Dev.* **1997**, *37*, 675–690. [CrossRef]
83. Hashimoto, Y.; Mori, M.; Kobayashi, S.; Hanya, A.; Watanabe, S.; Ohara, N.; Noguchi, T.; Kawai, T.; Okuyama, H. Canola and hydrogenated soybean oils accelerate ectopic bone formation induced by implantation of bone morphogenetic protein in mice. *Toxicol. Rep.* **2014**, *1*, 955–962. [CrossRef]
84. Ravnskov, U.; de Lorgeril, M.; Diamond, D.M.; Hama, R.; Hamazaki, T.; Hammarskjöl, B.; Hynes, N.; Kendrick, M.; Langsjoen, P.H.; Mascitelli, L.; McCully, K.S.; Okuyama, H.; Rosch, P.J.; Schersten, T.; Sultan, S.; Sundberg, R. LDL-C does not cause cardiovascular disease: a comprehensive review of the current literature. *Expert Rev. Clin. Pharmacol.* **2018**, *11*, 959–970. [CrossRef]
85. de Souza, R.J.; Mente, A.; Maroleanu, A.; Cozma, A.I.; Ha, V.; Kishibe, T.; Uleryk, E.; Budylowski, P.; Schünemann, H.; Beyene, J.; et al. Intake of saturated and trans unsaturated fatty acids and risk of all-cause mortality, cardiovascular disease, and type 2 diabetes: systematic review and meta-analysis of observational studies. *BMJ* **2015**, *351*, h3978. [CrossRef] [PubMed]
86. Booth, S.L.; Lichtenstein, A.H.; O'Brien-Morse, M.; McKeown, N.M.; Wood, R.J.; Saltzman, E.; Gundberg, C.M. Effects of a hydrogenated form of vitamin K on bone formation and resorption. *Am. J. Clin. Nutr.* **2001**, *74*, 783–790. [CrossRef]
87. Booth, S.L.; Tucker, K.L.; Chen, H.; Hannan, M.T.; Gagnon, D.R.; Cupples, L.A.; Wilson, P.W.; Ordovas, J.; Schaefer, E.J.; Dawson-Hughes, B.; Kiel, D.P. Dietary vitamin K intakes are associated with hip fracture but not with bone mineral density in elderly men and women. *Am. J. Clin. Nutr.* **2000**, *71*, 1201–1208. [CrossRef]
88. Knapen, M.H.J.; Drummen, N.E.; Smit, E.; Vermeer, C.; Theuwissen, E. Three-year low-dose menaquinone-7 supplementation helps decrease bone loss in healthy postmenopausal women. *Osteoporos Int.* **2013**, *24*, 2499–2507. [CrossRef] [PubMed]

89. Troy, L.M.; Jacques, P.F.; Hannan, M.T.; Kiel, D.P.; Lichtenstein, A.H.; Kennedy, E.T.; Booth, S.L. Dihydrophylloquinone intake is associated with low bone mineral density in men and women. *Am. J. Clin. Nutr.* **2007**, *86*, 504–508. [CrossRef]
90. Yoshida, M.; Jacques, P.F.; Meigs, J.B.; Saltzman, E.; Shea, M.K.; Grundberg, C.; Dawson-Hughes, B.; Dallal, G.; Booth, S.L. Effect of vitamin K supplementation on insulin resistance in older men and women. *Diabetes Care* **2008**, *31*, 2092–2096. [CrossRef] [PubMed]
91. Choi, H.J.; Yu, J.; Choi, H.; An, J.H.; Kim, S.W.; Park, K.S.; Jang, H.C.; Kim, S.Y.; Shin, C.S. Vitamin K2 supplementation improves insulin sensitivity via osteocalcin metabolism: a placebo-controlled trial. *Diabetes Care* **2011**, *34*, e147. [CrossRef] [PubMed]
92. Geleijnse, J.M.; Vermeer, C.; Grobbee, D.E.; Schurgers, L.J.; Knapen, M.H.J.; van der Meer, I.M.; Hofman, A.; Witteman, J.C.M. Dietary intake of menaquinone is associated with a reduced risk of coronary heart disease: the Rotterdam Study. *J. Nutr.* **2004**, *134*, 3100–3105. [CrossRef]
93. Fusaro, F.; Tripepi, G.; Noale, M.; Plebani, M.; Zaninotto, M.; Piccoli, A.; Naso, A.; Miozzo, D.; Giannini, S.; Avolio, M.; Foschi, A.; Rizzo, M.A.; Gallieni, M.; Vertebral Fractures and Vascular Calcifications Study Group. Prevalence of vertebral fractures, vascular calcifications, and mortality in warfarin treated hemodialysis patients. *Curr. Vasc. Pharmacol.* **2015**, *13*, 248–258. [CrossRef] [PubMed]
94. Iwamoto, I.; Takeda, T.; Ichimura, S. Effect of combined administration of vitamin D3 and vitamin K2 on bone mineral density of the lumbar spine in postmenopausal women with osteoporosis. *J. Orthop. Sci.* **2000**, *5*, 546–551. [CrossRef]
95. Nimptsch, K.; Rohrmann, S.; Kaaks, R.; Linseisen, J. Dietary vitamin K intake in relation to cancer incidence and mortality: results from the heidelberg cohort of the European Prospective Investigation Into Cancer and Nutrition (EPIC-Heidelberg). *Am. J. Clin. Nutr.* **2010**, *91*, 1348–1358. [CrossRef]
96. Fusaro, M.; Crepaldi, G.; Maggi, S.; Galli, F.; D'Angelo, A.; Calò, L.; Giannini, S.; Miozzo, D.; Gallieni, M. Vitamin K, bone fractures, and vascular calcifications in chronic kidney disease: an important but poorly studied relationship. *J. Endocrinol. Investig.* **2011**, *34*, 317–323. [CrossRef]
97. Shiraki, M.; Shiraki, Y.; Aoki, C.; Miura, M. Vitamin K2 (menatetrenone) effectively prevents fractures and sustains lumbar bone mineral density in osteoporosis. *J. Bone Miner. Res.* **2000**, *15*, 515–521. [CrossRef]
98. Rønn, S.H.; Harsløf, T.; Pedersen, S.B.; Langdahl, B.L. Vitamin K2 (menaquinone-7) prevents age-related deterioration of trabecular bone microarchitecture at the tibia in postmenopausal women. *Eur. J. Endocrinol.* **2016**, *175*, 541–549. [CrossRef] [PubMed]
99. Schmid, A.; Schmid, H. Rapeseed poisoning in wild herbivores. *Tierarztl. Prax.* **1992**, *20*, 321–325. (In German)
100. European Food Safety Authority. Analysis of occurrence of 3-monochloropropane-1,2-diol (3-MCPD) in food in Europe in the years 2009-2011 and preliminary exposure assessment. *EFSA J.* **2013**, *11*, 3381. [CrossRef]

101. Sauvaget, C.; Nagano, J.; Hayashi, M.; Yamada, M. Animal protein, animal fat, and cholesterol intakes and risk of cerebral infarction mortality in the adult health study. *Stroke* **2004**, *35*, 1531–1537. [CrossRef]
102. Yamagishi, K.; Iso, H.; Yatsuya, H.; Tanabe, N.; Date, C.; Kikuchi, S.; Yamamoto, A.; Inaba, Y.; Tamakoshi, A.; JACC Study Group. Dietary intake of saturated fatty acids and mortality from cardiovascular disease in Japanese: the Japan Collaborative Cohort Study for Evaluation of Cancer Risk (JACC) Study. *Am. J. Clin. Nutr.* **2010**, *92*, 759–765. [CrossRef]
103. Yatsuya, H.; Iso, H.; Yamagishi, K.; Kokubo, Y.; Saito, I.; Suzuki, K.; Sawada, N.; Inoue, M.; Tsugane, S. Development of a point-based prediction model for the incidence of total stroke: Japan public health center study. *Stroke* **2013**, *44*, 1295–1302. [CrossRef]
104. Nakazato, R.; Gransar, H.; Berman, D.S.; Cheng, V.Y.; Lin, F.Y.; Achenbach, S.; Al-Mallah, M.; Budoff, M.J.; Cademartiri, F.; Callister, T.Q.; et al. Statins use and coronary artery plaque composition: results from the International Multicenter CONFIRM Registry. *Atherosclerosis* **2012**, *225*, 148–153. [CrossRef]
105. Hirota, T.; Ieiri, I. Drug-drug interactions that interfere with statin metabolism. *Expert Opin. Drug Metab. Toxicol.* **2005**, *11*, 1435–1447. [CrossRef]
106. Singh, S.; Nautiyal, A. Aortic dissection and aortic aneurysms associated with fluoroquinolones: A systematic review and meta-analysis. *Am. J. Med.* **2017**, *130*, 1449–1457.e9. [CrossRef]
107. Cornett, E.; Novitch, M.B.; Kaye, A.D.; Pann, C.A.; Bangalore, H.S.; Allred, G.; Bral, M.; Jhita, P.K.; Kaye, A.M. Macrolide and fluoroquinolone mediated cardiac arrhythmias: clinical considerations and comprehensive review. *Postgrad. Med.* **2017**, *129*, 715–724. [CrossRef] [PubMed]
108. Ninomiya, T. Japanese legacy cohort studies: The Hisayama Study. *J. Epidemiol.* **2018**, *28*, 444–451. [CrossRef] [PubMed]
109. Kobayakawa, A. Healthy Life Should Be Gained by Yourself—Proposal on the Active Health Community. In *Proceedings of the 30th Memorial Lecture Meeting of Hisayama Town. Strategy of Prevention of Circulatory Diseases, Japan*; Shuppanbu, D.G., Teruo, O., Mastoshi, F., Ueda, K., Eds.; 1993; pp. 32–43. (In Japanese)
110. Hisayama Town. *Hisayama Town 60th Anniversary, Development of 8500 Towners, the Past and Future of Hisayama Town*; Kaichosha Publishing: Hukuoka, Japan, 2016. (In Japanese)
111. OECD. *Health at a Glance 2017: OECD Indicators*; OECD Publiahig: Paris, France, 2017. [CrossRef]
112. Sekikawa, M.; Tominaga, K.; Takahashi, H.; Eguchi, M.; Igarashi, H.; Ohnuma, K.; Sugiyama, H.; Manaka, H.; Sasaki, H.; Fukuyama, H.; Miyazawa, K. Prevalence of diabetes and impaired glucose tolerance in Funagata area, Japan. *Diabetes Care* **1993**, *16*, 570–574. [CrossRef] [PubMed]
113. Shirota, T.; Oishi, A.; Uchida, K.; Shinohara, A.; Uchida, K.; Kiyohara, Y.; Hujishima, M. Changes in nutritional status and nutritional intake among elderly residents of a community over a 10-year period: The Hisayama Study. *Jpn. J. Geriatr.* **2002**, *39*, 69–74. (In Japanese) [CrossRef]

114. Health and Nutrition Survey in Yamagata, Ministry of Health, Labour and Welfare, Japan 2000. Available online: https://www.pref.yamagata.jp/kenfuku/kenko/plan/7090015kenkoueiyouchousahome.html (accessed on 28 September 2020).
115. World Population Prospects 2017 Revision, United Nations DESA/Population Division. Available online: https://www.un.org/en/desa/world-population-prospects-2017-revision (accessed on 3 March 2021).
116. Morisaki, N.; Urayama, K.Y.; Yoshii, K.; Subramanian, S.V.; Yokoya, S. Ecological analysis of secular trends in low birth weight births and adult height in Japan. *J. Epidemiol. Community Health* **2017**, *71*, 1014–1018. [CrossRef]
117. Kajantie, E.; Osmond, C.; Barker, D.J.P.; Eriksson, J.G. Preterm birth–a risk factor for type 2 diabetes? The Helsinki Birth Cohort Study. *Diabetes Care* **2010**, *33*, 2623–2625. [CrossRef]
118. Lahti, J.; Räikkönen, K.; Pesonen, A.-K.; Heinonen, K.; Kajantie, E.; Forsén, T.; Osmond, C.; Barker, D.J.P.; Eriksson, J.G. Prenatal growth, postnatal growth and trait anxiety in late adulthood – The Helsinki Birth Cohort Study. *Acta Psychiatr. Scand.* **2010**, *121*, 227–235. [CrossRef]
119. Yamagishi, K.; Kitamura, A.; Kiyama, M.; Okada, T.; Sankai, T.; Imano, H.; Cui, R.; Umesawa, M.; Iso, H. Lifestyle and biomarkers as risk and beneficial factors of stroke in the circulatory risk in communities' study. *Jpn. J. Stroke* **2005**, *37*, 367–373. [CrossRef]
120. Markaki, I.; Nilsson, U.; Kostulas, K.; Sjöstrand, C. High cholesterol levels are associated with improved long-term survival after acute ischemic stroke. *J. Stroke Cerebrovasc. Dis.* **2014**, *23*, e47–e53. [CrossRef] [PubMed]
121. Tatematsu, K.; Hirose, N.; Ichikawa, Y.; Fujii, Y.; Takami, A.; Okuyama, H. Nutritional evaluation of an inter-esterified perilla oil and lard in comparison with butter and margarine based on the survival of stroke-prone spontaneously hypertensive (SHRSP) rats. *J. Health Sci.* **2004**, *50*, 108–111. [CrossRef]
122. GBD 2016 Stroke Collaborators. Global, regional, and national burden of stroke, 1990–2016: A systematic analysis for the Global Burden of Disease Study 2016. *Lancet Neurol.* **2019**, *18*, 439–458. [CrossRef]
123. Ning, X.; Sun, J.; Jiang, R.; Lu, H.; Bai, L.; Shi, M.; Tu, J.; Wu, Y.; Wang, J.; Zhang, J. Increased stroke burdens among the low-income young and middle aged in rural China. *Stroke* **2017**, *48*, 77–83. [CrossRef] [PubMed]
124. Fang, H.-Y.; He, H.-N.; Yu, D.-M.; Guo, Q.-Y.; Wand, X.; Xu, X.-I.; Zhao, L.-Y. Status and changes of edible oil consumption among Chinese residents. *China Foods Nutr.* **2016**, *23*, 56–58. (In Chinese)
125. Japan Dairy Association (J-milk), 2020. Available online: https://j-milk.jp/gyokai/database/index.html (accessed on December 23 2020).
126. Total Consumption and per Capita Consumption in Each Country, 2020. Available online: https://www.weblio.jp/wkpja/content/%E6%A4%8D%E7%89%A9%E6%B2%B9_%E5%90%84%E5%9B%BD%E3%81%AE%E7%B7%8F%E6%B6%88%E8%B2%BB%E9%87%8F%E3%81%A8%E4%B8%80%E4%BA%BA%E3%81%82%E3%81%9F%E3%82%8A%E3%81%AE%E6%B6%88%E8%B2%BB%E9%87%8F (accessed on 23 December 2020).

127. Okuyama, H.; Ohara, N.; Tatematsu, K.; Fuma, S.; Nonogaki, T.; Yamada, K.; Ichikawa, Y.; Miyazawa, D.; Yasui, Y.; Honma, S. Testosterone-lowering activity of canola and hydrogenated soybean oil in the stroke-prone spontaneously hypertensive rat. *J. Toxicol. Sci.* **2010**, *35*, 743–747. [CrossRef] [PubMed]
128. Oury, F.; Sumara, G.; Sumara, O.; Ferron, M.; Chang, H.; Smith, C.E.; Hermo, L.; Suarez, S.; Roth, B.L.; Ducy, P.; et al. Endocrine regulation of male fertility by the skeleton. *Cell* **2011**, *144*, 796–809. [CrossRef] [PubMed]
129. Oury, F.; Khrimian, L.; Denny, C.A.; Gardin, A.; Chamouni, A.; Goeden, N.; Huang, Y.; Lee, H.; Srinivas, P.; Gao, X.-B.; et al. Maternal and offspring pools of osteocalcin influence brain development and functions. *Cell* **2013**, *155*, 228–241. [CrossRef]
130. Payne, A.H.; Youngblood, G.L.; Sha, L.; Burgos-Trinidad, M.; Hammond, S.H. Hormonal regulation of steroidogenic enzyme gene expression in Leydig cells. *J. Steroid. Biochem. Mol. Biol.* **1992**, *43*, 895–906. [CrossRef]
131. Andersson, A.-M.; Jørgensen, N.; Main, K.M.; Toppari, J.; Rajpert-De Meyts, E.; Leffers, H.; Juul, A.; Jensen, T.K.; Skakkebæk, N.E. Adverse trends in male reproductive health: we may have reached a crucial 'tipping point'. *Int. J. Androl.* **2008**, *31*, 74–80. [CrossRef]
132. Iwamoto, T.; Nozawa, S.; Yoshiike, M.; Hoshino, T.; Baba, K.; Matsushita, T.; Tanaka, S.N.; Naka, M.; Skakkebæk, N.E.; Jørgensen, N. Semen quality of 324 fertile Japanese men. *Hum. Reprod.* **2006**, *21*, 760–765. [CrossRef]
133. Kameyama, T.; Ohhara, T.; Nakashima, Y.; Naito, Y.; Huang, M.Z.; Watanabe, S.; Kobayashi, T.; Okuyama, H.; Yamada, K.; Nabeshima, T. Effects of dietary vegetable oils on behavior and drug responses in mice. *Biol. Pharm. Bull.* **1996**, *19*, 400–404. [CrossRef]
134. Estimates of the Prevalence of Recognition Disorder in Aged Population, Cabinet Office, Japan. Available online: https://www.mhlw.go.jp/web/t_doc?dataId=80090000&dataType=0&pageNo=1 (accessed on 23 December 2020).
135. 3-CHLORO-1,2-PROPANEDIOL, Evaluations of the Joint FAO/WHO Expert Committee on Food Additives (JECFA), 2006. Available online: https://apps.who.int/food-additives-contaminants-jecfa-database/chemical.aspx?chemID (accessed on 23 December 2020).
136. Scandinavian Simvastatin Survival Study Group. Randomized trial of cholesterol lowering in 4444 patients with coronary heart disease: the Scandinavian Simvastatin Survival Study (4S). *Lancet* **1994**, *344*, 1383–1389. [CrossRef]
137. Matsuzaki, M.; Kita, T.; Mabuchi, H.; Matsuzawa, Y.; Nakaya, N.; Oikawa, S.; Saito, Y.; Sasaki, J.; Shimamoto, K.; Itakura, H.; J-LIT Study Group. Japan Lipid Intervention Trial. Large scale cohort study of the relationship between serum cholesterol concentration and coronary events with low-dose simvastatin therapy in Japanese patients with hypercholesterolemia. *Circ. J.* **2002**, *66*, 1087–1095. [CrossRef] [PubMed]
138. Mabuchi, H.; Miyamoto, S.; Ueda, K.; Oota, M.; Takegoshi, T.; Wakasugi, T.; Takeda, R. Causes of death in patients with familial hypercholesterolemia. *Atherosclerosis* **1986**, *61*, 1–6. [CrossRef]
139. Rosch, P.J. *Fat and Cholesterol Don't Cause Heart Attacks and Statins are Not the Solution*; Columbus Publishing Ltd.: Cwmbran, UK, 2016.

140. de Lorgeril, M. *Cholesterol Mensonges et Propagande*; Japanese, *!!! REPLACE !!!*, Ed.; Hamazaki, T., Translator; Japanese ed.; Hamazaki, T., Trans. Shinohara Shuppan Shinsha: Tokyo, Japan, 2009. (In Japanese)
141. Yoshiike, N.; Tanaka, H. J-LIT Area Controlled Follow-Up study. *Lipid* **2001**, *12*, 281–289. (In Japanese)
142. Okamura, T.; Tanaka, H.; Miyamatsu, N.; Hayakawa, T.; Kadowaki, T.; Kita, Y.; Nakamura, Y.; Okayama, A.; Ueshima, H.; NIPPONDATA80 Research Group. The relationship between serum total cholesterol and all-cause or cause-specific mortality in a 17.3-year study of a Japanese cohort. *Atherosclerosis* **2007**, *190*, 216–223. [CrossRef]
143. Sugiyama, D.; Okamura, T.; Watanabe, M.; Higashiyama, A.; Okuda, N.; Nakamura, Y.; Hozawa, A.; Kita, Y.; Kadota, A.; Murakami, Y.; et al. Risk of hypercholesterolemia for cardiovascular disease and the population attributable fraction in a 24-year Japanese cohort study. *J. Atheroscler. Thromb.* **2015**, *22*, 95–107. [CrossRef]
144. Okamura, T.; Kokubo, Y.; Watanabe, M.; Higashiyama, A.; Miyamoto, Y.; Yoshimasa, Y.; Okayama, A. Low-density lipoprotein cholesterol and non-high-density lipoprotein cholesterol and the incidence of cardiovascular disease in an urban Japanese cohort study: The Suita Study. *Atherosclerosis* **2009**, *203*, 587–592. [CrossRef]
145. Asayama, K.; Satoh, M.; Murakami, Y.; Ohkubo, T.; Nagasawa, S.; Tsuji, I.; Nakayama, T.; Okayama, A.; Miura, K.; Imai, Y.; et al. Evidence for Cardiovascular Prevention From Observational Cohorts in Japan (EPOCH-JAPAN) Research Group. Cardiovascular risk with and without antihypertensive drug treatment in the Japanese General population: participant-level meta-analysis. *Hypertension* **2014**, *63*, 1189–1197. [CrossRef]
146. Ogushi, Y.; Kobayashi, S.; Kurita, Y.; Yamada, T.; Abe, K. Verification based on the Guidelines for the treatment of hypertension. *Jpn. J. Med. Inform.* **2009**, *28*, 125–137. (In Japanese)
147. Irie, N.; Sairenchi, T.; Iso, H.; Shimamoto, T. Prediction of mortality from findings of annual health check-ups utility for health care programs. *Jpn. J. Public Health* **2001**, *48*, 95–108, In Japanese with English abstract.
148. Mori, H.; Ishiguro, K.; Okuyama, H. Hypertension in rats does not potentiate hypercholesterolemia and aortic cholesterol deposition induced by a hypercholesterolemic diet. *Lipids* **1993**, *28*, 109–113. [CrossRef] [PubMed]
149. Ueshima, H. Evaluation and counterplan for hypertension among Japanese-from NIPPONDATA. *Med Frontline* **1996**, *5*, 661–669. (In Japanese)
150. Hama, R. Editorial. Scientific evidence of hypertension guidelines 2019 is weak. Setting <130/80 mmHg as blood pressure lowering is risky. *Med. Check* **2019**, *19*, 104–109. (In Japanese)
151. Boffa, R.J.; Constanti, M.; Floyd, C.N. Hypertension in adults: summary of updated NICE guidance. *BMJ* **2019**, *367*, l5310. [CrossRef]
152. James, P.A.; Oparil, S.; Carter, B.L.; Cushman, W.C.; Dennison-Himmelfarb, C.; Handler, J.; Lackland, D.T.; LeFevre, M.L.; MacKenszie, T.D.; Ogedegbe, O.; et al. 2014 evidence-based guideline for the management of high blood pressure in adults: report from the panel

members appointed to the Eighth Joint National Committee (JNC 8). *JAMA* **2014**, *311*, 507–520. [CrossRef] [PubMed]

153. Umemura, S.; Arima, H.; Arima, S.; Asayama, K.; Dohi, Y.; Hirooka, Y.; Horio, T.; Hoshide, S.; Ikeda, S.; Ishimitsu, T.; et al. The Japanese Society of Hypertension Guidelines for the Management of Hypertension (JSH 2019). *Hypertension* **2019**, *42*, 1235–1481. [CrossRef]

154. Bakris, G.; Ali, W.; Parati, G. ACC/AHA versus ESC/ESH on hypertension guidelines: JACC Guideline comparison. *J. Am. Coll. Cardiol.* **2019**, *73*, 3018–3126. [CrossRef]

155. Look AHEAD Research Group; Wing, R.R.; Bolin, P.; Brancati, F.L.; Bray, G.A.; Clark, J.M.; Coday, M.; Crow, R.S.; Curtis, J.M.; Egan, C.M.; et al. Cardiovascular effects of intensive lifestyle intervention in type 2 diabetes. *N. Engl. J. Med.* **2013**, *369*, 145–154. [CrossRef]

156. Action to Control Cardiovascular Risk in Diabetes Study Group; Gerstein, H.C.; Miller, M.E.; Byington, R.P.; Goff, D.C., Jr.; Bigger, J.T.; Buse, J.B.; Cushman, W.C.; Genuth, S.; Ismail-Beigi, F.; et al. Effects of intensive glucose lowering in type 2 diabetes. *N. Engl. J. Med.* **2008**, *358*, 2545–2559.

157. Gerstein, H.C.; Miller, M.E.; Ismail-Beigi, F.; Largay, J.; McDonald, C.; Lochnan, H.A.; Booth, G.L.; ACCORD Study Group. Effects of intensive glycemic control on ischemic heart disease: analysis of data from the randomized, controlled ACCORD trial. *Lancet* **2014**, *384*, 1936–1941. [CrossRef]

158. Duckworth, W.; Abraira, C.; Moritz, T.; Reda, D.; Emanuele, N.; Reaven, P.D.; Zieve, F.J.; Marks, J.; Davis, S.N.; Hayward, R.; et al. Glucose control and vascular complications in veterans with type 2 diabetes. *N. Engl. J. Med.* **2009**, *360*, 129–139. [CrossRef]

159. Hayward, R.A.; Reaven, P.D.; Wiitala, W.L.; Bahn, G.D.; Reda, D.J.; Ge, L.; McCarren, M.; Duckworth, W.C.; Emanuele, N.V.; VADT Investigators. Follow-up of glycemic control and cardiovascular outcomes in type 2 diabetes. *N. Engl. J. Med.* **2015**, *372*, 2197–2206. [CrossRef]

160. Zoungas, S.; Chalmers, J.; Neal, B.; Billot, L.; Li, Q.; Hirakawa, Y.; Arima, H.; Monaghan, H.; Joshi, R.; Colagiuri, S.; Cooper, M.E.; et al. Follow-up of blood-pressure lowering and glucose control in type 2 diabetes. *N. Engl. J. Med.* **2014**, *371*, 1392–1406. [CrossRef]

161. Chalmers, J.; Perkovic, V.; Joshi, R.; Patel, A. ADVANCE: breaking new ground in type 2 diabetes. *J. Hypertens Suppl.* **2006**, *24*, 22–28. [CrossRef] [PubMed]

162. Araki, E.; Goto, A.; Kondo, T.; Noda, M.; Noto, H.; Origasa, H.; Osawa, H.; Taguchi, A.; Tanizawa, Y.; Tobe, K.; et al. Japanese Clinical Practice Guideline for Diabetes 2019. *Diabetes Investig.* **2020**, *11*, 1020–1076. [CrossRef]

163. Treatment Guide for Diabetes 2016-2017. The Japan Diabetes Society. Available online: http://www.fa.kyorin.co.jp/jds/uploads/Treatment_Guide_for_Diabetes_2016-2017.pdf (accessed on 24 December 2020).

164. The Japanese Council on Cerebro-Cardiovascular Disease. Comprehensive Risk Management Chart for Cerebro-cardiovascular Disease 2019. *Nihon Naika Gakkai Zasshi* **2019**, *108*, 1024–1074. [CrossRef]

165. American Diabetes Association. 1. Improving care and promoting health in populations: standards of medical care in diabetes 2019. *Diabetes Care* **2019**, *42* (Suppl. 1), 7–12. [CrossRef]
166. Hamazaki, T.; Okuyama, H.; Ogushi, Y.; Hama, R. Cholesterol issues in Japan–why are the goals of cholesterol levels set so low? *Ann. Nutr. Metab.* **2013**, *62*, 32–36. [CrossRef] [PubMed]
167. Pons-Rejraji, H.; Brugnon, F.; Sion, B.; Maqdasy, S.; Gouby, G.; Pereira, B.; Marceau, G.; Gremeau, A.; Drevet, J.; Grizard, G.; et al. Evaluation of atorvastatin efficacy and toxicity on spermatozoa, accessory glands and gonadal hormones of healthy men: A pilot prospective clinical trial. *Reprod. Biol. Endocrinol.* **2014**, *12*, 65. [CrossRef]
168. Ueki, K.; Sasako, T.; Okazaki, Y.; Kato, M.; Okahata, S.; Katsuyama, H.; Haraguchi, M.; Morita, A.; Ohashi, K.; Hara, K.; et al. Effect of an intensified multifactorial intervention on cardiovascular outcomes and mortality in type 2 diabetes (J-DOIT3): An open-label, randomized controlled trial. *Lancet Diabetes Endocrinol.* **2017**, *5*, 951–964. [CrossRef]
169. Okuyama, H.; Hama, R.; Ogushi, Y.; Hamazaki, T.; Uchino, H. Critical examination of the problems associated with the J-DOIT3 study and a proposal for its follow-up study, an intensified intervention in diabetics with hypertension and dyslipidemia. *J. Lipid Nutr.* **2018**, *27*, 30–38, In Japanese with English abstract. [CrossRef]
170. Prospective Studies Collaboration; Lewington, S.; Whitlock, G.; Clarke, R.; Sherliker, P.; Emberson, J.; Halsey, J.; Qizilbash, N.; Peto, R.; Collins, R.; et al. Blood cholesterol and vascular mortality by age, sex, and blood pressure: a meta-analysis of individual data from 61 prospective studies with 55,000 vascular deaths. *Lancet* **2007**, *370*, 1829–1839. [CrossRef]
171. Okuyama, H.; Hamazaki, T.; Ogushi, Y. New cholesterol guidelines for longevity (2010). *World Rev. Nutr. Diet.* **2011**, *102*, 124–136. [PubMed]
172. de Lorgeril, M. *Cholesterol, Mensonges et Propagande*; Thierry Souccar Editions: Vergèze, France, 2007.
173. Okuyama, H.; Hamazaki, T.; Hama, R.; Ogushi, Y.; Kobayashi, T.; Ohara, N.; Uchino, H. A critical review of the consensus statement from the European Atherosclerosis Society Consensus Panel 2017. *Pharmacology* **2018**, *101*, 184–218. [CrossRef] [PubMed]
174. Deol, P.; Kozlova, E.; Valdez, M.; Ho, C.; Yang, E.-W.; Richardson, H.; Gonzalez, G.; Truong, E.; Reid, J.; Valdez, J.; Deans, J.R.; Martinez-Lomeli, J.; Evans, J.R.; Jiang, T.; Sladek, F.M.; Curras-Collazo, M.C. Dysregulation of hypothalamic gene expression and the oxytocinergic system by soybean oil diets in male mice. *Endocrinology* **2020**, *161*, bqz044. [CrossRef]
175. Guasch-Ferré, M.; Liu, G.; Li, Y.; Sampson, L.; Manson, J.A.E.; Salas-Salvadó, J.; Martínez-Gonzále, M.A.; Stampfer, M.J.; Willett, W.C.; Sun, Q.; et al. Olive oil consumption and cardiovascular risk in U.S. adults. *J. Am. Coll. Cardiol.* **2020**, *75*. [CrossRef] [PubMed]

© 2021 by the authors. Licensee MDPI, Basel, Switzerland. This article is an open access article distributed under the terms and conditions of the Creative Commons Attribution (CC BY) license (http://creativecommons.org/licenses/by/4.0/).

www.ingramcontent.com/pod-product-compliance
Lightning Source LLC
LaVergne TN
LVHW072311090526
838202LV00018B/2263